I CAN'T HAVE CANCER, I HAVE CARPOOL!

I CAN'T HAVE CANCER, I HAVE CARPOOL!

Lessons on Beating Cancer While Being a Mom

Elizabeth Hodges

BOOKLOGIX®
Alpharetta, Georgia

The author has tried to recreate events, locations, and conversations from his/her memories of them. The author has made every effort to give credit to the source of any images, quotes, or other material contained within and obtain permissions when feasible.

Copyright © 2025 by Elizabeth Hodges

All rights reserved. No part of this book may be reproduced or transmitted in any form or by any means, electronic or mechanical, including photocopying, recording, or any information storage and retrieval system, without permission in writing from the author.

ISBN: 978-1-6653-0907-3 - Paperback
eISBN: 978-1-6653-0908-0 - eBook

These ISBNs are the property of BookLogix for the express purpose of sales and distribution of this title. The content of this book is the property of the copyright holder only. BookLogix does not hold any ownership of the content of this book and is not liable in any way for the materials contained within. The views and opinions expressed in this book are the property of the Author/Copyright holder and do not necessarily reflect those of BookLogix.

Library of Congress Control Number: 2024927453

⊛This paper meets the requirements of ANSI/NISO Z39.48-1992 (Permanence of Paper)

032125

*For my daughters, Mia, Lily, and Eliza—
the brightest stars in my orbit.*

Contents

Letter to the Reader	*ix*
1: The Diagnosis That Doesn't Have to Change Your Life *The Early Days and Weeks*	1
2: The Hardest Conversations *Telling Your Children and Family You Have Cancer*	17
3: Life in Technicolor *Traversing the Emotions of Unintentional Change*	27
4: Accepting Your Journey *Giving up the Life You Planned for the Life That Is Waiting*	43
5: When the Calvary Leaves *The Early Steps to Self-Sufficiency*	57
6: The Ultimate Conflict *Caring for Yourself While Caring for Your Family*	71
7: When the Dust Settles *The Infamous "New Normal" Begins*	83
8: From Toddlers to Teens to Everything in Between *The Effects of Your Cancer on Your Children*	93
9: Managing Your Relationship and Cancer *A Partner Makes You a Mother—and a Survivor*	105
10: Cancer and the Working Mom *Balancing Your Professional Career, Your Personal Life, and Your Disease*	121
11: The Journey Forward *An Unknowable Road, but You Have What It Takes*	133
Acknowledgments	*145*
Endnotes	*147*

Letter to the Reader

Dear Reader,

You must feel like you're on a roller coaster. One minute, your life seems on track as you juggle raising your family and numerous commitments. The next, your world turns upside down when you receive the shocking and terrifying news that you have cancer. Your future feels uncertain. Any cancer diagnosis breeds fear and sadness about how your role as a mother might change.

My eighteen-year journey with cancer has taught me that motherhood can be the strongest motivator to survive—and thrive. *I Can't Have Cancer, I Have Carpool!* will help you travel cancer's uncertain road by using motherhood as a source of strength on your disease journey. With honesty, grit, and grace, this book outlines what you'll face from diagnosis to survivorship, the lessons I learned, and how to use them to reshape your life as a stronger, more focused individual. Drawing on years of personal experience as both a stay-at-home mom and later a working mother, I share how I navigated the early days after my diagnosis through years of managing my health with chronic cancer.

I was thirty-eight years old when diagnosed with leukemia; I had three small children and, as the cliché goes, my whole life in front of me. Six weeks after my cancer diagnosis, doctors determined I had adult cystic fibrosis. Faced with the stark reality that I might not live to see my children grow up, I used motherhood as my anchor, raising my children from toddlerhood through high school and into college.

I wish I had a book like this when I first received my diagnosis. Fear was all I knew that fateful day eighteen years ago. I needed something to turn to—a book or a fellow survivor to help me cope with the overwhelming anxiety and flood of information from the very start. The internet offered obvious, helpful advice but very little that focused on the human experience of being both a woman and a mother.

I Can't Have Cancer, I Have Carpool! isn't about multitasking through an illness; it's about discovering how motherhood can empower you and restore your sense of control while facing your disease. After reading these pages, I hope you will replace sadness with strength, fear with information, and uncertainty with action as you navigate your cancer journey. After all, driving carpool is sometimes the best alternative to letting cancer drive your life.

1

The Diagnosis That Doesn't Have to Change Your Life

The Early Days and Weeks

I have cancer.
I have cancer.
I have three small children, and I have cancer.
    Like a recording stuck on repeat, the words kept replaying in my mind as I sat in the emergency room. They spun endlessly on an imaginary hamster wheel, hoping for a place to stop. But doctors had just confirmed my cancer, so there was no stopping the truth.
    For women on the wrong end of these fateful words, you remember when you heard them. You recall the place, the time of day, and the people you were with. You felt tossed in the air, and your once-scripted life landed on the floor like scattered pieces of paper. Cancer threatens to shatter and unmoor your life instantly, casting you adrift in a direction you cannot control. And this, as a mother, feels unimaginably frightening.
    I understand because I have stood where you stand now.

MY DIAGNOSIS

Sitting in the airport departure lounge, I could practically smell the beach—our family was so ready for spring break. My husband, Alex, glanced at our five boarding passes, motioning for my three small daughters and me to join him in the cattle herd boarding the plane. Our twin daughters squirmed in their double stroller while pawing at the release clasps, trying to free themselves. My oldest dangled a toy in their faces to distract them from their confinement.

Airports are not the place you usually associate with cancer. Instead, they often bring anticipation of a new destination or experience. I, however, began a vastly different journey on March 6, 2006.

As we shuffled to join my husband in line, my cell phone rang unexpectedly in my pocket. Glancing down, I wondered who could be calling and saw my doctor's phone number. I had been waiting for blood test results from a lingering low-grade fever and headaches I couldn't shake. Mildly sick for months, I started seeing an infectious disease specialist to get to the bottom of recurring colds and other unexplained health issues. I foolishly believed my latest symptoms came from a newly formed allergy to coffee. I actually thought my lifelong love of java had suddenly made me ill.

Answering the phone, I joked with my doctor before he could say a word, "No matter what you say, I'm going to Florida!" We usually had a comfortable, easy banter, so I assumed his call would confirm my suspicion that I was indeed allergic to coffee. It seemed so plausible.

Immediately, I detected something different in my doctor's voice. He wasted no time cutting to the chase.

"Where are you?" he asked urgently.

"I'm at the airport; I'm about to depart," I said as I pushed the stroller forward, inching closer to the jet bridge. Alex looked at me quizzically, wondering why I was on the phone as our brood filed toward the plane. I mouthed my doctor's name.

"What's going on?" I asked, cradling the phone to my ear

while bending over to release our impatient twins from their stroller. "Did you get my blood results?"

"Yes. I did," my doctor responded, "and some numbers have come back really high. Your white blood cell count is off the charts." He sounded panicky.

I stopped unbuckling the girls and stood up, wondering if I had heard him correctly. "What do you mean 'high'? How high?" I asked, recalling somewhere that an elevated white blood cell count indicates severe illness.

My doctor's words came at me fast. "Your white blood cell count is over seventy-seven thousand. The normal range is around five to eleven thousand. It might be leukemia. I want to get your blood retested immediately because the results could be wrong. I need you to get to an emergency room as soon as possible."

Like a radio dial in my head slowly turning down the volume, the noise in the terminal began to fade. I felt my limbs go cold as I stepped out of line and walked to the window.

"Did you say 'leukemia'?" I asked quietly, not wanting others, nor myself, to hear the words. My heart thumped as my head began spinning.

"It could be. Again, the results might be wrong. That's why I want to get you retested immediately," my doctor responded, sounding more nervous.

Foolishly, almost desperately, I asked, "Does this mean I can't go to Florida?" Subconsciously, I knew the answer as soon as I posed the question.

"You can, but you must go straight to an emergency room the minute you land and get your blood drawn. And if it's leukemia, you'll have to come right back to Atlanta," he explained, continuing to sound panicky. "I don't recommend you do that. I've contacted the emergency room here and told them to expect you."

And then, I got panicky.

I hung up and turned to my husband, frantically waving at him to get out of line. Confused, he swiftly maneuvered the stroller and our daughters over to me. I croaked, half crying, that we had to leave. Now. Somewhere in my explanation of what my doctor told me, I said the word leukemia.

"What did you say?" Alex asked, also not believing what he heard. The twins danced around us—happy to be out of the stroller—but our oldest daughter grew suspicious of the unfolding drama.

"I might have leukemia," I whispered, gasping for air as I paced back and forth. "We have to go to the hospital immediately."

Exiting the airport became our first taste of what life with cancer and children would soon be like. Fear and confusion reigned as I tried to remain calm for my family. We spent excruciating minutes trying to get our squirming twins back into their stroller while telling them that we weren't going to Florida, but not saying exactly why. My husband moved expeditiously as my panic rose with each passing minute.

As we half ran through the concourse, Alex repeatedly asked me exactly what my doctor had said on the phone, convinced I had misunderstood him. I, too, wanted to believe it was a mistake. I just needed to get to the emergency room as fast as possible to prove it. But there, deep within me, where the truth flowed like a steady, unstoppable current, I knew. Something was terribly wrong.

Time moved like molasses as we stopped at baggage claim to organize our luggage delivery to the house. My daughters played on the stationary baggage carousel while my husband spoke with the airline customer service agent. I stood to the side, scared and speechless. My eyes darted nervously between my girls as I grew increasingly impatient. I wanted to bolt from the airport and go to the hospital myself.

Once in the car, we raced home as I called the babysitter to meet us while I fielded endless questions from our daughters, careful not to use the word cancer. After a fly-by drop-off of the kids, Alex and I continued to the emergency room, not speaking as we sped down the highway. What could we say? The possibility of what lay ahead felt incomprehensible.

Within minutes of checking in, a nurse swiftly escorted us to a room with a door—no flimsy curtain between patients for me. Cancer already had its privileges. I crawled up on the examination table, the crinkly white paper shifting underneath me.

Another nurse entered, drew my blood, and told me I would receive the results within an hour. Mentally, I continued grasping the slimmest hope—maybe, just maybe, there had been an error. I alternately prayed, cried, and stared at the clock on the wall before me. Its cold, matter-of-fact face glared back, daring me to look. The more I looked, the slower it moved. I called my pastor and left a message, "Can you call me as soon as you get this?"

Alex sat nearly motionless in one of the two red plastic chairs in front of me with his arms crossed over his chest as if to contain the flood of emotions building inside him. I don't remember what we said to each other in those sixty minutes before my life forever changed. I reached a point when I wished the doctor would never enter—never open the door to my new reality. Perhaps I could remain suspended in time in that white-walled room with the examination table, ticking clock, and two rigid seats.

I can still picture the young physician quietly entering the room an hour later, his dark hair gelled in perfect formation. He wore a crisply ironed white lab coat with his name stitched on the pocket. Holding a single piece of paper, he tried to hide the concern etched on his face—but I knew. Before the doctor could speak, I sucked in my breath and asked, "Is it leukemia?" He winced slightly at my question, then nodded. The doctor shared that my white blood cell count had risen substantially. There was no question: I had cancer.

Stifling the waves of sobs rising within me, I listened as he said I would be admitted to the hospital immediately to begin treatment. I could not go home, see my daughters, or pack a bag. When I asked how long I would remain there, the young physician told me six weeks. Six weeks. I thought of my girls and could feel my panic rising once more.

I turned to my husband as the sobs I tried to hold back now flowed uncontrollably. Tears streamed down my face as I struggled to say anything. Alex started to cry.

"Please stop," I choked through my tears. "Please. I will not survive this if you are not strong. I'm not sure if I can do this." Alex wiped his tears while nodding, the gravity of what I said sinking in.

At that moment, I didn't know if I would live or die. But I did know I would never return to my old life. A new journey had begun for me. But this time, it was not a trip I wanted to take.

Maybe I should've known something was wrong. Sure, numerous symptoms pointed to leukemia, but they also could have been a hundred other things. Who actually believes they have cancer? Persistent morning headaches made me think I had developed an allergy to coffee. Or, maybe I contracted my lingering low-grade fever from the kids and couldn't shake it. Yes, I was thinner than ever, but I worked out regularly. I felt tired, but no more than usual. Tiredness comes in many forms when you're a mom. It all seemed so explainable—until it wasn't. A doctor once told me, "Leukemia is like a snake in the grass; it sneaks up out of nowhere and bites you." Nothing could have been more true.

NAVIGATING THE EARLIEST DAYS AND WEEKS

Memories of the early hours and days following my

diagnosis remain crisp and clear. Fear flooded every ounce of my being. It felt so all-consuming I could practically taste it. I wasn't ready to die. And what about my children? Cancer doesn't just throw a wrench into your life; it also disrupts their world. You think you must get through this, not just for yourself, but for them.

But where do you begin when first diagnosed? As the floodgates of feelings and information fling open, you're suffering from understandable confusion and grief. My journey had just started, and already I felt adrift in a powerful current.

The time drifted past midnight as Alex and I waited in the emergency room for a bed to become available in the hospital. Not understanding the intricacies of my disease, I expected to be moved to a regular hospital room. But after an hour, a nurse transported me in a wheelchair to the bone marrow transplant unit. Bone Marrow Transplant? I stared in disbelief upon seeing the sign above the door. No one could enter this hospital wing without scrubbing their hands and donning a surgical mask, sterile gown, and shoe covers. I wondered what it was about my leukemia that required such protective measures. The sanitary environment and stringent hygiene rules felt like another nail hammered into the coffin containing my former life. The irony was inescapable; I went from an airport—the germ center of the universe—to a bacteria prevention bubble in less than twelve hours.

The nurse wheeled me to my room and told me that a hematology oncologist would be coming to meet me. I couldn't believe a physician was working so late. But given the bombshell that had hit my life hours before, I had countless questions, with my mortality topping the list.

I anticipated a stereotypical gruff doctor—overly intellectual, using words I had never heard before and, honestly, I didn't want to hear. Instead, a calm, quiet man later entered my room, wearing khakis and a button-down shirt. He was an older man with gray hair at his temples and small silver-framed glasses perched on his nose. His name slid off your tongue—Henry Holland.

Dr. Holland sat down leisurely, holding a small notepad and pen, making it hard for me not to feel at ease. He began by asking me a few questions about my health history. For a fleeting moment, I thought this was it! I could finally explain that I could not possibly have leukemia based on my symptoms. I imagined he would stop me midsentence and agree, saying that this had all been a big mistake: I didn't have leukemia. He would apologize and announce that I could leave. We would all have a good chuckle and go home tired but happy.

Instead, he listened patiently, scribbling notes while nodding his head. After reviewing every detail of my recent symptoms, he put down his pen and notepad. Slowly, Dr. Holland explained the type of leukemia I likely had and what would happen to me. In the dimly lit hospital room at one o'clock in the morning, I finally got the details I had dreaded but needed to hear. I had acute myeloid leukemia (AML) that would require intensive chemotherapy followed by a bone marrow transplant. He planned to use highly aggressive chemotherapy to destroy the leukemic cells in my bone marrow, then rebuild it with a marrow transplant from a donor. My chances of survival were 50/50. I could not leave the hospital during this time and was only allowed brief visits from my daughters.

Dr. Holland explained that despite my dire diagnosis, one glimmer of hope remained. He believed I had a slight chance of having a different type of leukemia—a chronic form—that he wanted to confirm with more bloodwork and a bone marrow aspiration. This chronic form did not require grueling treatment or a transplant, just daily medication. But, given my preliminary test results, he dismissed this as a slim possibility.

After answering a few more of my questions, Dr. Holland asked the nurse for an antianxiety medication to help me rest. As he left the room, Dr. Holland paused at the foot of my bed, looked me in the eye, and gently said, "We're going to get you better." For a second, I felt hopeful that it could be that easy, but deep down, I knew he couldn't promise me anything.

There is no more fearful time in your cancer journey than the day of your diagnosis and the weeks immediately following with confirmation of your condition, formation of your medical team, and discussion of treatment regimens. As information stormed my world, almost blinding me with its ferocity, I felt like I needed a roadmap outlining how to navigate my life from the earliest moments. Sure, countless online articles contained information on my leukemia along with suggestions on what to ask my doctor about the disease and treatment plan. However, very little focused on the human side of the experience, especially as a mother. Where did I begin? My world had shattered, and I had no idea how to start picking up the pieces surrounding me and my family.

So here is where we begin with the lessons I learned eighteen years ago. I hope they function as *your* roadmap for navigating the early days and weeks as a patient and a mother. Some suggestions might resonate with you; others might not. Remember, a cancer diagnosis doesn't have to change your life entirely if you begin by knowing where to start and what to expect.

✓ **Accept That Life Will Be a Fog**

Accept that you will understandably not think nor act clearly in the first weeks after your diagnosis. While I remember intricate details of the earliest hours and days, memories of my life after I left the hospital are hazy, fragmented glimpses of time. I do not have clear recollections of when I woke, slept, or how I spent my days. As I grappled with my new reality, I struggled to string concrete thoughts together—about anything. Now I understand this was my mind's way of sheltering me from the physical and emotional onslaught I experienced. Expect the fog (and its best friend, exhaustion) and know it will evaporate as your path forward becomes clear with your treatment plan and you gain your footing (sadly, the exhaustion will not evaporate).

✓ **When the Help Swoops In, Allow It**

Once you have informed extended family, friends, and neighbors, you'll find that everyone wants to help you after your diagnosis. As offers of assistance swoop in, allow them; just don't be the one to manage the onslaught. Your spouse, family member, or friend should begin by planning and organizing everything concerning your children, such as coordinating their daily schedule, playdates, afterschool activities, sports, etc. Other friends and neighbors who offer to help can cover different aspects of your life, including running errands or arranging meals for your family. These people should know your personality, family schedule, and personal preferences so they can organize these in an efficient manner that doesn't require your input or approval.

If you choose to keep your diagnosis private for personal reasons or to shield your children, consider who will be part of your Tribe (I will discuss this later) and who can aid you and your family early on. Oncology social workers affiliated with your oncologist's office, the American Cancer Society, or online providers such as CancerCare.org offer good resources for help.

✓ **Relinquish the Reins of Motherhood, For Now**

Just as people offer to help, you may struggle with allowing them to do so. Before cancer, you were the Superwoman in your house: you skillfully managed everything from A to Z. Now, the challenge of caring for yourself and managing your disease while raising your family feels overwhelming. You're conflicted as you relinquish much of what you want to do for your children versus what you should do for yourself.

But on this journey, know that you don't have to sacrifice being a good mother. You will find the balance between caring for yourself and being a loving mom. Society has falsely conditioned mothers to believe they must give 100 percent to their families at all times; anything less means falling short of an unrealistic standard. After your diagnosis, you may not be able to give 100 percent of your energy, but whether it's 40 percent, 20 percent, or even 1 percent, it's sufficient. What you give your children during these early days and weeks will be welcomed, loved, and *enough*. Hand over the reins if possible; you'll get them back before you know it.

✓ **Whom Will You Tell?**

Later, I will talk more about telling your children, but one of the first big questions after diagnosis will be whether to inform people you have cancer. This decision usually splits evenly between those who decide to share and those who don't. While I am a live-out-loud, tell-the-world-everything kind of person, many are not. Bottom line, it's your choice.

You may decide, for example, that only close family members, specific coworkers, and your children's teachers should know. Carefully explain your condition and ask that this not be shared with anyone; then assume it will be. It's normal for your news to get out without your consent. Just be prepared. Establish an agreement with those aware of your cancer regarding the message you want to share with others about your illness. A lack of a cohesive explanation might result in questions overwhelming you like a tsunami. Having to clarify information about your disease gets exhausting.

Only months after sharing my diagnosis widely, I wished I had not told as many people as I did. Acquaintances I barely knew reached out or approached me in public to ask how I was doing, showing incredible kindness. Repeatedly explaining my disease and sharing my progress wore me down despite their genuine concern. Not their fault—it was mine. I should have kept the circle of people who knew my story much smaller. Give careful thought to this before the news of your disease gets out.

✓ Who Are Your Eyes and Ears?

Meeting your oncologist for the first time feels daunting. It is one of those doctors you thought you would never have to encounter. Repeatedly seeing them for check-ups and in-depth discussions about your treatment progress and next steps can trigger a range of intense emotions. For this reason, in the early days and weeks, try not to see any doctor without an advocate. This person can be your spouse, significant other, family member, or friend. Choose the right person to be an extra set of eyes and ears. Whether they act as note-takers, hand-holders, or question-askers, their role is crucial.

Carefully think about how you and your advocate want to prepare before these visits. Do you want to research your disease online before speaking with your oncologist so you can ask informed questions? Treatment options can be confusing. Do you prefer your doctor to lead the discussion? Understand what feels right for you. Whatever the case, if you or your advocate develop a habit of carefully recording information early, it will help you feel more confident in each stage of your treatment journey.

I suggest having a written list of questions before each appointment. Have your phone ready to record the visit because no matter how clear-headed you think you feel or how well your advocate takes notes, you might want to review something you heard. Recording your meetings allows you to listen to the information again when your mind is calmer.

✓ **Understand How You Want to Receive Information**
Juggling the influx of data from all areas of your life will feel taxing immediately after your diagnosis. For this reason, understand how you want to receive information. For example, hearing that your high school son is failing physics one minute and then details on your cancer treatment plan the next is a lot to absorb. Despite your disease, life will go on, so know what you can and cannot process.

Consider dividing information into medical and personal buckets. I adopted the "information is power" mindset when managing the medical aspects of my life. The more I understood about my leukemia, the better I felt, even if it terrified me. However, I also knew I could not simultaneously process updates from my children's teachers about how, for instance, one of my daughters struggled in math and needed a tutor. My husband and a small cadre of friends managed this so I could focus solely on my treatment and communication with my doctors.

It's easy to think you can still handle everything as smoothly as you did before your diagnosis, and maybe you can. But if it all feels overwhelming, communicate what information you can and cannot handle in the earliest days and weeks—you'll be glad you did.

✓ **You May Not Sleep**
No surprise here. Sleep will be elusive as every conceivable thought races through your mind each night. I advise you not to battle the beast of sleep deprivation with everything you're facing early on. Countless options exist to help you sleep, from prescription medications to over-the-counter solutions, allowing you to rest during this critical time. Your oncologist can recommend or prescribe what

you need and should be knowledgeable about the available options.

I started a prescription sleep aid soon after my diagnosis and continued to take it for at least six months. Admittedly, I worried about becoming dependent on sleeping pills and not being able to sleep without them. When I expressed this to my oncologist, he replied, "That's the last thing you need to be concerned about right now. You have bigger fish to fry." Well said.

✓ **You Will Be Down**

No surprise here, either. You will likely be incredibly down, dare I even say depressed, from the beginning. Understand how you want to handle the inevitable sadness and grief that accompanies any diagnosis—no matter the severity. Take the necessary steps to address this and work with your doctor to find effective solutions. You do not need to suffer when you're already facing so much. Options to combat depression or regularly feeling low include prescription medication, meditation, support groups, therapy, or natural supplements (check to ensure that these do not impact your chemotherapy).

Because the response to my treatment, and therefore my survival, remained unknown for many months, my doctor recommended I take an antidepressant. However, the first prescribed medication made me incredibly sleepy and zoned out—not my desired response. I subsequently spent several months not taking an antidepressant and then needed one as I suffered from PTSD from all the stress much later.

✓ **Resist the Urge to Control: Take it Day by Day**

As your oncologist outlines your disease and treatment plan early on, you might be searching for something to anchor yourself in the chaos of your new reality. On my first night in the hospital, I sat poring over the pages of a medical encyclopedia my husband brought me from home while waiting for my oncologist. I figured I could start learning about my leukemia right away. Foolishly, I believed that if I understood every aspect of my disease, I could wrestle it to the ground—control it. Instead, I sat drowning in pools of fear and confusion when I should have first listened to my doctor's expertise.

Cancer treatment often follows a prescribed step-by-step approach to achieving a cure or remission. Your medical team will outline the course of action and the results they hope to see at each stage. You have to take it one step at a time—far easier said than done. Patience over your situation will be short. You're a mother, for God's sake, you don't have time for cancer. Resist the urge to understand everything all at once.

As you adopt this one-day-at-a-time approach, try to continue activities you enjoyed before cancer. Even better, do these with your children to spend quality time together. The sooner you learn to engage in distractions to rest your hyperactive mind, the better off you will be.

KEY REFLECTIONS

Almost everything changes when cancer changes everything. From the initial shock of diagnosis to navigating treatment and managing daily life amidst uncertainty, the journey is one of immense challenges and demands resilience. While a cancer diagnosis is profoundly significant, it doesn't have to derail one's life completely.

Develop your roadmap for navigating the early days and weeks. Much of it is acceptance and the importance of communication, support systems, and self-care in coping with the physical, emotional, and practical aspects of living with cancer. Despite the difficulties, you can navigate this challenging early period with support and a focus on what truly matters.

2

The Hardest Conversations

Telling Your Children and Family You Have Cancer

Just as no one wishes to hear that they have cancer, no one relishes delivering the news that they have cancer—not to loved ones, especially your children. It feels unfair, and frankly, the timing always stinks. Cancer often strikes right when your kids, no matter what age, are experiencing an intense phase of needing you. Whether it be separation anxiety, potty training woes, the first day of elementary school, middle school drama, or the high school social circus, cancer loves to enter the room when the I need my mom light flashes brightest. You really can't have cancer—you have carpool and countless other important, even mundane, things to do for your family. Your children need you.

But now, the paradigm will flip, and you must be cared for as dutifully as you care for your children. Others may not completely take over your role, but they will step in to help. And this—this temporary shift of parenting to your spouse, family, or friends—challenges you to your very core.

On my third day in the hospital, Alex brought two of our three daughters to visit me. One of the twins stayed home with a cold. We wedged ourselves into a tiny nurse's office given to us for our reunion and privacy. Dressed in their sterile gowns and facemasks, my daughters walked in cautiously, clutching homemade get-well cards while eyeing the cramped surroundings. They hugged me gently, taking care not to bump my IV pole. My two-year-old twin, Eliza, circled the room and asked questions about everything around her.

"What's that for?" pointing to my IV pole.

"What's that for?" pointing to a computer on the nurse's desk, wanting to touch it.

"Why are you wearing that, Mommy?" pointing to my hospital gown.

How had I missed the delicate golden color of Eliza's hair and her devilish smile? Had she always been this curious? My six-year-old, Mia, suspicious of everything happening to me, laughed nervously at her sister's bubbly questions but remained silent and wide-eyed as she clung to Alex. When did she grow another two inches? I wondered. Seeing them produced tears of joy and sadness—they never looked so beautiful. My heart ached, knowing the visit would only last a few minutes.

We decided not to tell our daughters about my diagnosis that day. Their young age and the complexity of my disease and treatment felt more than they, let alone I, could handle. Instead, I asked questions about what they had been doing at home.

Home. My rightful place now felt remote and far away.

They shared the small details of their lives, as children so wonderfully do. My girls described the toys they played with (Barbies), the TV shows and movies they watched (Toy Story), and the bubble baths they enjoyed. It stabbed me to hear it. Already, I missed the regular, routine pattern of our lives. Why had I taken it for granted? I thought I had paid attention to the details of the beautiful mosaic that made up our lives, but in that moment, I realized I hadn't.

In a blink, our visit drew to a close. My husband started putting on the girls' coats and shuffled them toward the door. I yearned to rip off my face mask and dash out of the hospital with them. Trying to remain upbeat, I helped my husband and said—lied—that I would be out of the hospital soon. Miraculously, no one started crying as we walked down the hallway to the large, mechanical doors of the bone marrow transplant wing. After passing through them, my daughters turned to wave as the doors inched their way closed. Sobs rose and remained perched in my throat as I waved back. I turned and walked back to my room, trying to silence my sobs—grateful, for the first time, for my face mask.

When would I go home? I wondered as I entered the bleak room where I now lived.

Even worse, would I go home?

TELLING YOUR CHILDREN

Mothers often want to shelter their children from difficult news or challenging situations. It's natural to want to hide your cancer diagnosis. In truth, unless you have very young children, it may be hard, if not impossible, to hide the disease from your family. The sudden emergence of extended family, neighbors, and friends bombing in to help quickly alerts them that something is amiss.

Deciding how to tell your children feels fraught with emotion and complexity. Frankly, the perfect way does not exist. You do your best to consider the right time, how to explain your illness, what to expect, and countless other details. But, by being honest and forthright early, in an age-appropriate way, you pave a path to express how you feel physically and emotionally from the very beginning. The more you include your children in your journey, the healthier the experience will be for all of you.

Consider these ideas before talking to your family:

✓ **Talk to a Professional First**

Before talking to your kids, you may want to speak with a therapist specializing in child psychology. You might ask for an oncology social worker at the hospital or clinic, at the start or during your ongoing treatment, to be assigned to your case to assist you with the right words and timing. Even if you do not seek assistance from a professional, practice what you will say and anticipate your child's questions. This preparation will help you stay calm and focused on the points you want to convey without succumbing to your emotions or theirs—much easier said than done. If your spouse or partner must tell your children because you are in the hospital or simply unable to, discuss beforehand what they will say (again, seek help from a licensed professional).

✓ **Consider When and How to Tell Your Children**

There's no perfect moment to talk to your children. Honestly, when is the right time to tell anyone you have cancer? You might choose to wait to get test results back to confirm details of your disease before informing your kids. If possible, have the conversation when you feel calm-ish, and neither you nor your children feel distracted, tired, or stressed. Think about the right time of day and allow plenty of time for discussion. Decide if you want to tell them yourself or prefer to have someone with you, such as your spouse, partner, or a valued family member. This option might be best if your emotions run (understandably) high and another person can remain calm and focused. View the first conversation as a starting point that begins an ongoing process of gradually giving your children small, relevant pieces of information and reassurance. Consider using simple, straightforward language to describe your disease. Of course, the age of your children will also dictate how and what to say, as I detail below. Allow the conversation to be directed by your children's reactions and the questions they ask. While your kids may inquire about what will happen, keep information relevant and focused on your current situation rather than what might occur in the future. Be prepared for them to react in their own way.[1]

✓ **Telling Little Ones**

My twin daughters were two years old at the time of my diagnosis, so I ruled them out of any detailed explanation of my leukemia. I figured it would be easier to tell them mommy was sick versus trying to describe my cancer and attempting to answer the ensuing questions. My six-year-old, however, was a mature girl who could sniff when something was awry. Our social worker advised us to share the facts with Mia at the appropriate time and in a simple, direct way: I had cancer and would have to go to the doctor often. They would do everything they could to help get me well. While she asked a few questions about the word "cancer," the experience went as planned. And I didn't lose it as I feared.

If you decide to tell your younger children, remember that toddlers and preschool children might feel insecure when their daily lives change because a parent becomes less available. They could sense your anxiety and become anxious themselves. Use clear and honest language to reassure your kids that, although you will need to be away for appointments or treatment, you love them and will be OK. Even if they cannot comprehend fully, your tone of voice will reassure them. We often forget that children are resilient and can handle disruptions better than expected. Nonetheless, make arrangements for them to spend regular time with loving adults who can focus on their needs during this time.

Elementary children will notice disruptions to household routines, your mood and any physical changes. Unfortunately, these changes can happen quickly, so ongoing conversations will assist when fear develops—both yours and theirs. Share with your children how much their love comforts you; allow them to do things they believe are helpful (even if they aren't).

Remember that on many days, just keeping your eyes open despite crippling fatigue will be your one remarkable feat of the day. There will also be times when you cry so many tears you could mop the floor. Your kids might be scared by this, but truthfully, you feel scared too, so why not draw a picture about it, read a funny book together, or play a game that gets both of your minds off the situation? Then, go take a nap.

On other days, your energy will be high, and you will feel good. Be patient if your children forget about your cancer and act out or resist being helpful. Relish these moments—as strange as that sounds—when motherhood feels like it used to! Make it a *Let's Pretend Mom Doesn't Have Cancer Day* and enjoy.

- ✓ **Telling Older Children**

Your older children will likely understand your cancer diagnosis but may be more fearful. But remember that school-aged children are not miniature adults. They also need information in a straightforward, simple manner. If necessary, share that they will not get your cancer; they bear no responsibility for causing it, nor could they have done anything to prevent this from happening. Understandably, your kids will also be concerned about what to expect in the future and how it might affect them. No senior in high school, for example, wants to hear their mother has cancer. It hurts all of you.

If you feel comfortable, share your treatment plan with your children and, if you choose, be honest about your prognosis. Always remember that even with your family, your health history remains yours. Whether you share every detail or just an overview is entirely your decision.

Explain that your treatment regimen could result in changes to the family routine. If they express interest, bring older children to a chemotherapy session or doctor's visit so they understand your experience. They might inquire about genetic links to your disease and the chances of getting it when they're older. Encourage them to ask your oncologist or care team questions, which, hopefully, they will find helpful and reassuring.

Consider whether you want your older children to share news of your cancer with other people, which may be impossible to avoid. Again, your health is your business. The last thing you want is a pesky phone call from a parent you barely know asking questions because they heard about you from their kid. Of course, you can't blame your child—just be prepared.

Bottom line, try to lay the groundwork for an open line of communication with your children—a way for them to come to you with their questions, needs, and fears. Some may blame themselves for your disease, no matter what age. While heartbreaking to hear, your best—your only—approach is to be as honest and open as possible about how your illness works.

✓ **Telling Extended Family**

As with any disease, cancer is just as hard for family members to come to terms with as it is for you. Nonetheless, you likely need your family to help when the bottom falls out. The night of my diagnosis, I remember calling my parents and saying the word that felt so foreign in my mouth—leukemia. Given our close relationship, I considered this call one of the worst I had to make. They dropped everything and drove ten hours to care for my girls the next day.

My dad immediately came to the hospital to see me the minute they arrived. Upon entering my room, I started to cry. Unlike other times in my life, I knew my father couldn't fix this. I had never seen him look more tired, frightened, and yet ready to help. So, I asked him to just sit with me, knowing there was little else he could do. We watched TV, talked, or read the newspaper together while the endless parade of doctors and nurses filtered through my room. My father felt like a calm wind in my medical tornado.

Informing your family will likely invoke immediate offers of assistance. But, with this good might come the not-so-good. My parents, for instance, provided tremendous support during my hospital stay and after I returned home. They knew how to care for my girls, who felt happy and secure with them, and I will be forever grateful. However, as time went on and the reality of my situation set in, things began to change slightly.

Slowly, my mother wanted to take over and fix what she perceived had "caused all this." Consciously, my mom knew she couldn't cure me, but she began identifying things she thought needed correcting. For example, she believed the rug in my twins' bedroom had a "chemical smell" (it didn't), which, according to my mother, could have contributed to my cancer. It needed to go. She reasoned the cleaning products I used in my house certainly weren't doing me any good. They, too, needed to go. And maybe I needed to take more vitamins. Over time, I grew frustrated with her focus on trivial things while avoiding the elephant in the room.

This frustration reached a breaking point one night when my mother and I stayed up late talking. While she discussed carpool logistics and the weekly meal plan, I contemplated my mortality. As she quietly chattered on, I slid from the couch to the floor as a loud guttural moan poured out of me. The all-consuming sadness over my situation burst like a dam. I sobbed uncontrollably. My mother came to my side, nervously asking, "What can I do? How can I fix this?" And that was precisely the point. My mom couldn't fix my cancer; nothing she did would cure my leukemia. I realized my mother coped with her fear by staying busy around my house.

Like me, she was afraid I would die. Doing things mitigated her sadness, even if it bothered me. Sitting on the floor, I carefully explained that I didn't care about tossing out a rug, cleaning supplies, or discussing family logistics. Those things meant little with cancer staring me in the face. We cried and shared more about our fears regarding the tremendous challenge I faced. My mother and I learned a lot about each other that night, even if we processed our grief in vastly different ways.

✓ **The School Connection**

If you think it is appropriate (and it probably is), you should notify your children's school of your diagnosis. Informing the school will allow teachers and administrators to assist you and your family through this trying time. The way I viewed it, I had volunteered for enough school events and classroom parties that it was our turn to ask for help.

My husband coordinated a meeting between the school counselor and my daughter's teachers to discuss my situation. He carefully explained my disease, what lay ahead, and how it would impact me. Alex shared that we had informed our oldest daughter and asked them to keep this in the strictest confidence out of respect for her. We expected my news would still likely spread throughout the school community but recognized the risk was worth the extra support we needed. Specifically, my husband and I immediately wanted to know if teachers began to notice behavioral or academic changes.

As expected, many learned of my situation. But, what happened after was nothing short of miraculous as countless people offered to make a meal, watch my children after school, or drive them wherever needed. I accepted many of these offers and allowed the love surrounding my daughters to buoy them while I managed my cancer storm.

KEY REFLECTIONS

Just as no one wishes to hear that they have cancer, no one relishes sharing that they have cancer, not with loved ones or people in their inner orbits. Still, this difficult conversation can create a tender moment and a lasting bond.

No matter whom you tell, be your authentic self with a simple and clear message: you have cancer, for which no one is to blame and which is not contagious to anyone. Seeking professional guidance in this process might ease the confusion, complications, and significant emotional charge of delivering news no one wants to say or hear.

These hard conversations come with consequences: by sharing your story, you share some of your emotions and sensitive information. Remember that you can use this vulnerable moment to create the attitude and mood that will surround you and your family to the best of your ability. We teach people, not just in this moment but throughout our lives, how to treat us, and you can use the sharing of your personal life to shape the life you want to live. Because of you and your message, the people you love and those who cooperate with you can become informed individuals, hopeful souls, passionate advocates, or whatever you help them to be.

3

Life in Technicolor

Traversing the Emotions of Unintentional Change

Unintentional change is unwelcome, and many feelings ignite after an unexpected life event like cancer. You will experience a long list of emotions as you move through your cancer journey. As they flood in, some will be predictable, and others will surprise you with their intensity and unexpected onslaught. You may swing from sadness that you may not live to be the mother you envisioned to immense relief that you have a family to love and support you during this time. There may be jealousy surrounding your spouse's good health or your friends' cancer-free lives. One day might bring elation from favorable test results, only to be followed by frustration over the long course of treatment ahead. No matter the case, no one wants to face these emotions of unintentional change.

Days after my diagnosis, still in the hospital, I ventured out of my room to stretch my legs. Pushing my IV pole along the nearly deserted hallways, I tried not to look into the other rooms but couldn't resist. I saw only a few patients, with most keeping their curtains drawn. I heard soft voices from hushed televisions in each quiet room. Nurses moved like purposeful swans in and out of each with few facial expressions. They experienced this every day—caring for people diagnosed with some of the most challenging and often deadly forms of leukemia.

I passed a young Asian woman pushing her IV pole with gusto. Clearly wanting to stretch her legs also, I noticed her bald head covered by a stylish knit cap. Her expressive eyes revealed the beauty hidden behind her face mask. Despite her circumstances, she confidently strode past me while talking on her cell phone with an "I've got this" attitude.

I didn't share her confidence and struggled to believe everything would work out. The nurses often reminded me, "Attitude is everything" when fighting leukemia. I fought to muster an ounce of positivity, let alone an optimistic outlook.

As I moved farther down the hall, a close family friend called my cell phone to check in on me.

"How are you?" he cautiously asked as I rattled past the nurse's station.

"Meh," I replied, "I'm neither here nor there."

"You must feel like you're on a rollercoaster," he said empathetically.

I stopped when I heard this. My friend's statement hit me like lightning, capturing exactly how I felt. It felt so true: one moment I rose, hopeful and cautiously optimistic about my chances for survival. Then I would careen downhill, riding out of control with fear while being thrashed from side to side with anger and sadness, only to come to a complete stop of uncertainty. I rode a constant emotional rollercoaster of the worst kind. But then again, so did every single person in that leukemia wing.

The emotions you experience on your cancer journey will indeed feel like a rollercoaster, with ups and downs that amplify every moment. This heightened emotional intensity throws you into a vivid world where everything seems magnified, as if living in Technicolor. You notice *everything* around you—the beep on the machine dispensing your chemo, the electric blue sky on a sunny autumn day, the swish of your daughter's dress in a dance recital, or the sound of your son's kick of a soccer ball.

My life in Technicolor felt almost electrified as I became intensely aware of my thoughts and feelings about everything and everyone around me. My world seemed to buzz as I pondered my existence and everything in it daily. Each experience triggered a corresponding emotion, making me happy, mad, sad, or glad at every turn. In one way, we should always live with a heightened consciousness that drives our perception and appreciation of the world. And yet, moms with cancer would happily relinquish this Technicolor experience to live cancer-free. Give us a predictable and, dare I say it, boring life instead—no colorful, intense emotions needed. But this is not your path. Instead, you must learn to face—dare I say, accept—the many emotions you will encounter.

THE EMOTIONS OF UNINTENTIONAL CHANGE

Reaction to your cancer will generate an alphabet soup of feelings ranging from anger, fear, frustration, jealousy, and sadness over being the sick wife and mother to happiness and relief that you are still here. I experienced all of this and more. If I am honest, my feelings also included resentment. Resentment of my husband for his excellent health and the seemingly long life ahead of him plagued me. It brought me immense grief that I might die long before he did. With that came jealous thoughts over who he might marry and that she, not I, would become the mother to my children and share all the special moments that would soon come. I wondered who would and would not make a perfect replacement for me. I secretly hoped he would never remarry should I die, but simultaneously feared that my kids would be without the guidance of a loving mother.

Alternately, I would sometimes feel overwhelmed by the simple joy of being alive. I loved listening to my children giggle or sing while playing. I noticed the precise curl of my daughters' hair or the lilt in their voices when they asked me a question. My life seemed to buzz with hyperawareness as everything radiated a glow that demanded attention. And then, this bliss would disappear for no reason, and I fell into deep pools of sadness. My family witnessed it all—the full range of my experience, with its highs and lows, fully on display.

Some emotions you encounter will fall into predictable buckets. Others will surprise you with their intensity and sudden appearance when you least expect it. Tears of happiness or sadness might fall while you push toddlers on a swing or teach your teenager to drive. Sometimes, explaining these feelings on the fly ("Why are you crying, Mommy?") can be tricky, especially without the luxury of a place to compose yourself. The challenge becomes how to process these emotions while maintaining your fragile mental state. Your kids want to see a strong woman who embraces life and is eager to celebrate it with them. However, they may be just as scared as you about what is happening.

Being open about your feelings will help you and your children travel the normal yet bumpy road of unintended emotions. Finding the balance between when to be strong and when to be vulnerable develops over time. How you physically feel or appear will also dictate how you react on any given day. So, along with the expected shock following your diagnosis, here are some common emotions you will likely experience:

Fear—Beyond Normal

By now you know the most intense emotion you will experience immediately following your diagnosis will be fear. Cancer's relentless grip causes mothers to simultaneously fear death while also being terrified of facing their new reality. They want to be there for their family but have little idea how life might look going forward. You think of nothing but the future and what might happen.

Sitting on the windowsill of my hospital room, I stared out the dusty window and watched children playing on the playground below. The sound of a heater hissed nearby while a machine beeped quietly behind me. Outside, I noticed parents perched near their kids, casually watching while chatting with their friends.

Sadness and jealousy consumed me as I watched the children run, skip, and jump in the late afternoon sunshine. I could hear their voices through the window. Or was it my own daughters' voices echoing in my mind? I found myself wanting to smash the window and swoop down to that sacred space like a condor, assuming my rightful place with the other parents. I craved pushing my girls on a swing, not sitting in a hospital room waiting to hear if I would live or die from incurable leukemia.

My thoughts were interrupted when my oncologist, Dr. Holland, and his assistants entered my room. I noticed their slight smiles. Then I dismissed it, thinking I misread their reactions. There's not much smiling in a bone marrow transplant wing. Instead, life hangs by a thread in each room as transplants are among the most dangerous procedures a cancer patient will undergo.

Slowly, I moved from the windowsill to my bed. Everyone took a seat around me in the cramped space. A nurse wedged in to grab my vital signs and check the beeping machine before scurrying out as if she knew it was time for The Talk.

The Talk involves confirming with a newly diagnosed patient what form of cancer they have, the treatment, and the prognosis. Initially, Dr. Holland suspected Acute Myeloid Leukemia (AML), the most fatal type of leukemia. I had prepared myself for confirmation of AML. Instead, Dr. Holland shuffled a stack of lab reports, looked me in the eye, and stated that he had good news. He shared that while he initially believed I had AML, my bone marrow aspiration results revealed I actually had chronic myelogenous leukemia (CML). CML is a slow-growing, chronic form of the disease that progresses over many years and requires a vastly different treatment protocol. Dr. Holland told me that if I was going to get leukemia, this was the one to get. I guess I had hit some lucky cancer jackpot.

Only years before, CML had been almost as deadly as AML, with only a 30 percent survival rate after five years. A revolutionary new oral medication had transformed these survival rates and turned a once-fatal cancer into a chronic disease, with many patients living an average lifespan. There was one catch: you had to respond positively to the oral medicine to survive. If not, the only option was a bone marrow transplant, and I already knew what that entailed. The news made me happy but still uneasy. I had one question for my oncologist: "Will this medicine keep my leukemia away?" I asked him—not wanting to use the word cure. It felt like asking about a cure would be tempting fate.

"No. It is not a cure," Dr. Holland said as if reading my mind. "What we know from experience is your leukemia may come back, depending on how you respond to the medication," he added cautiously, trying to sound hopeful.

"When? When might it come back?" I probed.

"In about seven years, maybe ten," Dr. Holland stated matter-of-factly.

I nodded while discreetly tapping my fingers on my leg,

counting how old my daughters would be in seven years. According to his calculations, if the medication didn't work, my oldest daughter would be thirteen, and my twins nine years old when my CML returned, likely worse and more deadly.

"But," the doctor added, "this is a new medication, so we are learning a lot. Your response to the medicine could last much longer than that."

My thoughts bounced up and down like a yo-yo. One minute, immense relief washed over me that I didn't have an acute form of the disease; the next minute, my mind crashed down on death and no guarantees.

"Please, God, just let me live to see them graduate," I prayed silently, as fear surged through me so intensely I could almost taste it.

Every form of cancer requires extensive testing to determine the scope of the disease and approach to treatment. Visits to the oncologist, blood tests, scans, and biopsies combine to form a clear picture of your condition while spinning just enough unpredictability to upset your apple cart of calm. Then fear swoops in, always hovering and impossible to ignore, demanding to know what will happen.

Everyone told me that fear was completely normal. For me, fear felt not only normal but also ever-present. Over time, I learned to be comfortable with it as it ebbed and flowed throughout my survivorship. I found it impossible to escape, like a dark rain cloud that followed me wherever I went. Even when things on the ground went well, I would look up to see that tireless, hovering rain cloud.

Fear and uncertainty about my leukemia sent me down rabbit holes of the worst kind. My mind became stuck on an endless loop of questions: *What if this happens? What if that happens? Will I die? Will I live?* Over and over, I spun on my mental hamster wheel of fear that turned faster each time I looked at my children, asking myself countless unanswerable questions.

Slowly, over many months, if not years, my new mental soundtrack contained the phrases: *You are not crazy; being scared is normal,* and *Everything will be OK.* I'll share tips on how I learned to accept my fear later, but reaching this point required a lot of practice and patience. Taking care of myself and putting fear in its rightful place each day to be present with my children became paramount. On many days I succeeded, but on just as many, I failed.

Sadness—the Ultimate Puppet Master

In addition to fear, I also felt sad. Tremendous sadness. Deep sadness. Feeling sad and even hopeless is an expected fallout, and, like fear, sadness envelops everything. Everywhere you turn, reminders lurk. Your children become daily taps on your shoulders of the tremendous stakes you face.

The need to be patient intensifies sadness. Cancer treatment demands time and patience, two things in short supply for a mother. Life already feels dramatically upended, and now you must wait to see what will happen. You realize that no matter how much you might have complained about your life before cancer, it seemed far better than what you now face. And that generates incredible sadness.

Sadness also silently fuels or masks other emotions— anger, jealousy, and even rage. I discovered that it operates like a puppet master hoisting the strings of different feelings up and down. After my diagnosis, I moved from doomsday predictions about what could happen (fear) to an almost Zen-like acceptance of my fate (contentment). I thought about whether I would live or die ten times a day (worry). Envious of my husband and his good health (jealousy), I would mock

I Can't Have Cancer, I Have Carpool!

him whenever he hesitated to take even an ibuprofen if he didn't feel well. "Want to walk a mile in my shoes?" became my go-to statement to get him to shut up if he complained about something plaguing him. It was mean and vindictive, borne out of profound sadness over my situation. If I wasn't crying, at least I could sling cruel verbal arrows to make myself feel better. It rarely worked and only served to make a sad situation worse.

With time, sadness usually softens and evolves into acceptance. It takes fortitude and patience for this process to blossom fully. Yet, you possess more resilience than you think. Ultimately, you are greater than your sadness, and you will not and cannot let your cancer journey be defined by it.

Anger—It Eats Away at You

I admit I have some anger issues, often triggered by traffic, feeling overwhelmed by my kids, running late, or a host of other reasons. I've actively worked on managing my reactions and finding healthier ways to cope over the years, but cancer did nothing to help my problem. Anger may arise at any time throughout treatment and survivorship. I wish I could tell you I am no longer prone to anger after more than eighteen years of living with chronic leukemia. Truthfully, anger has become the most challenging emotion I've experienced.

Anger may surface once the reality of your situation sinks in and treatments disrupt your family's routine. Oddly, I became mad at myself for not appreciating all the little things I thought annoyed me as a mother *before* my diagnosis. The perpetual cleaning up, laundry, organizing the next meal, playdate, or carpool felt like a dream life I desperately wanted back. I never imagined I would love driving carpool as much as I did until I got leukemia.

Anger with cancer often involves other people, including

how family members and friends react to your diagnosis. They may say too much or not ask at all. Some may cease contact out of fear of saying the wrong thing, which will make you mad. And sad. And don't get me started on the folks who believed they had the answer to getting me well. Like those people who insinuated that if I just ate the right foods, consumed herbs, or meditated more—you name it—it would cure my cancer. Or if I removed certain toxic things in my home, life, or routine, I would get better. Of course they meant well, but I needed to focus first and foremost on my medical treatment before accepting extraneous advice.

The one statement I heard from some that often irritated me most was four simple words: "I am so sorry." Please understand me: everyone who said this compassionate sentiment offered it with profound love and concern for my well-being. No one wants to see someone stricken with cancer. My issue with these words was 100 percent my problem; maybe you can relate. The statement made me feel like an incapable woman and mother navigating a death sentence. Angrily, I thought to myself, *I don't need your sympathy. I can handle this cancer; my life isn't over.* I crafted other retorts in my head but never stated them, including, *That's what you say when someone has died. The last time I checked, I'm not dead yet.* And on and on. My inner anger knew no bounds.

Anger may also stem from your struggle to cope with the side effects of cancer and its treatment, including fatigue, pain, nausea, hair loss, sleeping problems, or a thousand other things. These can make even the happiest person feel irritable. Ironically, the angrier you get, the unhealthier you feel. The emotions you experience as your cancer persists are often worse than the physical carnage it may inflict on your body. You see, cancer feeds not just on your body but on your mind. Your body is a remarkable organism capable of healing.

However, your mind can generate thoughts that can take over your life. Awareness of this will help you move away from anger and toward healing.

Worry—Not the Same as Anxiety

Worry and anxiety are both powerful emotions linked to cancer, but they are not the same. Indeed, the most challenging part of managing your disease may not be the cancer itself, but the worry and anxiety of living with it. You're probably saying right now, "I don't *choose* to worry about my cancer. It just happens." And this is true, sort of. You may tell yourself you aren't worried: *Everything will work out. Breathe, just breathe.* But cancer affects the body, and on any given day, even without cancer, you may experience inexplicable aches or pains. A pulled muscle in your torso? Your mind goes to liver or lung cancer. Swollen lymph nodes in your neck could mean your cancer is back, worse, or something else. It could also be an upper respiratory infection. You try to ignore these things while repeating to yourself, *Calm down.* But, what if you're wrong, and it is a new symptom? Anyone would worry under these circumstances, which also generates anxiety.

According to *Psychology Today,* the difference between worry and anxiety is, "Worry tends to be more focused on thoughts in our heads, while anxiety is more visceral in that we feel it throughout our bodies."[2] When we worry, our specific concerns generate our thoughts, which we can resolve by problem-solving. An example of a worrying thought is, "If I don't take my medication at a certain time, it might not work as effectively as it should." Once you identify the problem and arrive at the solution—to take your medicine at the prescribed time—you will likely move on from this thought and diminish worry.

I've cried buckets of tears worrying about a resurgence

of my leukemia. Whatever inexplicable symptom I experienced—ambiguous pain, unexplained bruising, or weight loss—became a sign that my cancer had resurged and I would descend into hell again. Each time, I whipped out my laptop to research all the iterations of my symptoms, imagining the worst. Sometimes I would call my oncologist's office to discuss my concern. Then, with accurate information or a visit to my doctor, I would slowly calm down enough to honestly assess my situation.

Health anxiety, like worry, is natural and entirely normal for a cancer survivor. When we experience anxiety, however, our thoughts might be more vague. They can linger for extended periods and can negatively impact our lives. An example is persistently thinking something will go wrong every time you see your oncologist or visit your clinic for labs, treatment, or a simple check-up. As a result, you experience anxiety that causes your body to react negatively. The physical reactions caused by anxiety, however, can be more intense than worry. Someone with anxiety may experience symptoms such as tightness in the chest, an increased heart rate, rapid breathing, headaches, trembling, gastrointestinal problems, or trouble sleeping. [3]

Seeing friends or family might trigger anxiety. You feel anxious that someone might say something to make you feel unhinged. Even worse, they could say something in front of your children that you prefer not to discuss openly. You can likely list many things that fuel your anxiety, and simply being told not to worry won't make it go away. You might try to reassure yourself that everything will be fine even as that small voice within you, the one you want to murder, keeps asking: *Are you sure everything will be OK? How do you know?* Which only drives more stress and anxiety.

Learning how to manage your worry or health anxiety

often comes after months or even years of practice. You get better at knowing what to do when you feel these emotions about your disease. I now know how to seek information on a given symptom to alleviate my worry. Reading clinical data or research on disease progression or specific conditions no longer scares me. The internet has become my friend, not my foe. When it all becomes too much, and I feel anxious, I employ some of the suggestions below. If needed, I'll call my doctor or nurse practitioner or schedule an office visit to alleviate anxiety. Why suffer when you can get an answer to ease your feelings?

USING YOUR EMOTIONS FOR GOOD

Dealing with the emotions of a cancer diagnosis requires a lot of patience and, frankly, a pull-yourself-up-by-the-bootstraps approach to navigating them. Your genuine feelings deserve respect from you and everyone around you, including your family. Ultimately, however, managing your emotions comes down to your own will and effort. This process begins with accepting the normalcy of your feelings, which ebb and flow over time. Practice self-compassion as you adjust to your situation and find the tools you need to handle the intense, Technicolor-like emotions and roller-coaster of feelings.

Many options exist to help you, but some to consider include:
- ✓ **Find Fellow Survivors**

Despite genuine attempts by family and friends to provide emotional support, sometimes it might not be enough. In my case, I had exhausted my husband and those closest to me with my need for my feelings to be heard and understood. I wanted someone to live in my world for five minutes to understand my fear and desperation. But realistically, how can anyone but a fellow cancer survivor possibly know how you feel?

Instead, find someone or a group of people walking the same road as you. Rather than a family member trying to solve what they can't possibly understand, find a support group who can. They offer emotional support from fellow survivors and help you feel less alone. Support groups are everywhere—online, at your local clinic, oncologist's office, or hospital. They can be a lifeline. Maybe you need more than one: a regular in-person group and an online support forum where discussions flow freely, and you can join in when you have disease-specific questions.

When I couldn't find a CML support group in my area, I formed one. Meeting with fellow CML survivors, even our small but mighty group of five people, helped me feel validated. I drew immense strength from sitting with survivors in the same room as we shared stories and compared side effects and treatment options. We discussed the different stages of remission and our mental health while swapping tips on various topics related to our shared journey. After each meeting, I left feeling happy: I wasn't alone! I returned home better equipped to focus on being a mother and spouse—something the entire family needed.

✓ **Own What You Are Experiencing and Take Action**

If cancer makes you feel powerless and emotionally vulnerable, take back control by doing what you can to master the chaos swirling around you. Taking the initiative to call your doctor or care team with questions or scheduling your next visit feels empowering. Learn a non-scary way to search the internet for answers. Small steps on the big road to recovery begin with you. Over time, you will figure out whom to call and what to do to manage everything relating to your disease. You will discover that each twinge is not a significant cause for concern, but learning how to get answers on your own is essential.

Sadly, everyone reaches a point of oversaturation with cancer—even you. Once again, it is not that people don't care about you or your situation; life simply moves on. The difference is that your family and friends can walk away from your disease, but you cannot. And that's where your resilience kicks in. As the empowered driver of your wellness journey, you decide how you want to manage everything. Feeling strong enough mentally and physically to attend your next doctor's appointment yourself? Go for it. Want to go to chemo, your next scan, or bloodwork alone? Do it. Want to understand your disease better? Open your laptop. Learn how to bolster yourself with facts about your condition and allow clinical data to light your path, no matter how anxiety-provoking. Information is power when it comes to cancer.

Throughout all of this, part of your arsenal might be medication or another method to help tame your emotions. Consider enlisting a therapist as another member of your care team to discuss how to process your feelings. Find the combination of things that works for you and take action. Medication to treat my anxiety and mild depression and regular sessions with a therapist shored me up. Slowly, over months and after much work, I trained myself to stop cycling on fear—or whatever the day's emotion. I discovered there was a time for my feelings and a time to live my life and raise my family.

✓ **Repeatedly Tell Yourself That All Feelings Are Normal**

Navigating the ups and downs of life with cancer and its complex emotions is a serious challenge, but you can do it. Remind yourself each day that your feelings are normal, have a purpose, and can be managed, not just tamed. Derive strength from solving this puzzle and continually ask, *What do I need?* Be gentle with yourself. You'll lose your shit occasionally as you figure it out. That's OK. Start over the next day and the next day after that.

KEY REFLECTIONS

Ultimately, we want to channel our emotions to fuel our progress in fighting cancer. Learning to handle your feelings and needs early will build the muscle needed to support yourself and strengthen you. Know that the Technicolor existence will fade, and the rollercoaster ride will smooth out. Find your method of managing challenging emotions and allow good feelings to flourish as much as possible so you can enjoy your children now. Appreciate that cancer has taught you to live in the moment. Don't let emotions get in the way of noticing life's highs and lows, the big and small moments with your family.

4

Accepting Your Journey

*Giving up the Life You
Planned for the Life That Is Waiting*

As mothers, we often try to limit the unpredictability and uncertainty of parenting. Having a daily, weekly, or monthly schedule helps us create order and maintain a sense of control. Before cancer, I believed I could meticulously plan my life. I thought that with a solid plan, I could handle any challenges that came my way. I naively assumed that things would generally follow my almighty design. Sure, life would bring its share of surprises, but nothing I couldn't manage. I carefully crafted my days and our family's activities, balancing my career with raising our children. It all seemed so doable.

And then the universe laughed at my plans. Every. Damn. One.

Six weeks after being diagnosed with CML, I again sat listening to a doctor diagnose me with a life-threatening condition. The phone call, intended to discuss the possibility of a bone marrow transplant to cure my leukemia—a treatment I desperately hoped for, given my young age—turned into the revelation of something vastly different. Before this call, my oncologist had sent my health history to a leading pulmonary hospital to determine if my lungs were healthy enough to survive a transplant. Instead, I listened as a pulmonologist from the hospital explained that, while reviewing my lung history, his team had discovered unusual damage caused by years of unexplained illnesses. Digging deeper, they found the reason.

"We think you have adult cystic fibrosis (CF)," the pulmonologist stated matter-of-factly as if he said it a hundred times a day.

"Wait. I'm sorry, what did you say? I have what?" I asked, pushing my cell phone to my ear as if that would change what he said.

"I said we think you have adult cystic fibrosis," the doctor said calmly. "The health history and scans of your lungs that Dr. Holland sent over lead us to believe it's true. But we need a few more tests to confirm. Are you able to come to our clinic anytime soon?"

I stared at my laptop and the minutiae on my desk, unable to process his words. What was he saying to me? I realized I had yet to recover from the shock of my first diagnosis. "I thought this call was to discuss if I could get a bone marrow transplant and be cured of CML. How is this possible?" I asked, my voice and anxiety rising with the idea of being diagnosed with another chronic, life-threatening disease. "There must be a mistake. I cannot have cystic fibrosis."

"I'm sorry. I know this is shocking. But, we have every reason to believe it's true," the pulmonologist said, again sounding so calm.

"Do you understand that I was just diagnosed with leukemia? This can't be right." I frantically hoped he would shuffle the test results in front of him and agree with me that there had been a mix-up. Someone else had adult CF, not me. His bad.

"Listen, if you hadn't been diagnosed with CML, we might never

I Can't Have Cancer, I Have Carpool!

have found this. So, in a sense, we're lucky. It certainly explains your recurring lung infections since you were a child and numerous bouts with pneumonia. Luckily, we think it's a mild, rare form of the disease," he finished, softening his approach as if the leukemia part of my life had finally registered.

This time, my body didn't go cold with fear, and my brain didn't descend into a fog. Another disease on top of leukemia? I thought. What were the odds? Instead of learning if I could be cured of one life-threatening disease, doctors discovered I had another. I felt oddly resigned. Shocked and speechless but resigned nonetheless.

As the doctor described what I could expect and the treatment required for adult CF, my mind drifted off, unable to absorb more detailed medical information. I turned away from my desk and looked out the window of my office. I noticed the sun shining outside and recall thinking, "Wow. The sun really does rise each day." I had begun to doubt this law of nature. When you receive terrible news, your world feels so dark you think maybe it won't happen, and your life remains permanently dim.

As I continued staring at the sunshine blanketing my yard, I marveled at how I could be diagnosed with two life-threatening chronic diseases within six weeks. It felt unjust. Why me? I asked myself. But then again, why not me? Life goes on, both the beautiful and the not-so-beautiful. And just as the sun rises each day, I know that anything can happen at any moment. Life rarely goes according to plan. The more we try to control it, the less likely we are to get what we want. It's like sand in your hands; the tighter you squeeze, the more it slips away.

The moment doctors confirmed adult cystic fibrosis, they immediately ruled out a bone marrow transplant for CML. A complete cure for my leukemia was now off the table. Instead, I would continue to take a daily chemo pill to treat my disease. The addition of cystic fibrosis, however, brought more medications to my routine, including inhalers, frequent antibiotics, and daily lung clearance exercises I needed to perform with a machine. There is no cure for adult cystic fibrosis.

Like everyone on chemotherapy and now CF medications, I suffered horrible side effects—crushing fatigue, digestive issues, headaches, weight gain, sleeplessness—you name it, I experienced it. Fortunately, the targeted CML medication offered a high probability of inducing remission. Unfortunately, I had to take it every day for years, maybe the rest of my life. It resembled a daily vitamin, but rather than making me healthy and pumping me with essential nutrients, this drug is toxic to my liver and leaves me feeling sick if not taken correctly. I worried about the long-term impact on my body and whether this drug could cause another form of cancer.

I worried too about cystic fibrosis as it is a degenerative lung disease that literally and figuratively takes your breath away without proper care. Adult CF requires rigorous attention to treatment as the disease causes thick, sticky mucus to build up in the lungs, digestive tract, and other areas of the body. Even with mild CF, failure to preserve lung function can produce hospitalizations, the need for even more medicines, and long-term health issues.

My health was clearly under assault. I felt my ability to manage my family slipping away. I envisioned myself on an island with sharks circling, while in the distance, safe on solid ground, my family waved for me to come back and be their rock. But how could I be a strong mother with so many compromising health issues?

But what choice did I have? I could continue to be concerned about the many what-ifs I faced or accept my fate. I experienced great emotion and pain in abandoning my idea of how motherhood would unfold. Of course, I knew life would produce its expected share of ups and downs, painful moments, and uncertainties. But, I never expected how much cancer, and now adult cystic fibrosis, would alter my approach as a mom. It forced me to accept a new reality and rethink everything. With two life-threatening diseases, I had less time to devote to my children and certainly less energy. Planning my future was replaced by focusing on the present. This change forced me to plan my days around caring for myself, my children, and not much else—a significant change indeed.

THE LIFE THAT IS WAITING FOR YOU: FINDING YOUR NEW HORIZON

Any cancer diagnosis feels like a horrible fate. While filled with crushing emotions and physical demands, cancer also presents an opportunity. It doesn't have to derail your life completely. But that has to be your decision, and you then have to take the pivotal steps to ensure you execute your new life, cancer and all. William Faulkner said it best: "You cannot swim for new horizons until you have the courage to let go of the shore."

But what if the effort to reach your new horizon (life after cancer) feels overwhelming and painful? Assume it will be—and then dig deep to muster the strength to move in the direction of getting well. How do you overcome the fear surrounding each doctor visit and check-up? Go to them to get through them. How do you confront the trauma surrounding frequent scans, blood work, and test results? Face them with all the courage you can. Tired of the daily medications you have to swallow? Grab the glass of water. Each endeavor you undertake to treat your cancer becomes another step toward being there for your children. You move toward your new horizon as a cancer survivor. It's unfamiliar, exhausting, and frightening. But remember, beyond that horizon, your family and a new life await you.

This focused intention to move through your cancer experience with strength and courage gets easier with time and more commonplace in your life. It is a new life for sure, but maybe, just maybe, as the captain of your ship, you determine your destiny (with a little help from medical science). And boy, does this make you stronger. Each time I went to the doctor armed with questions about my progress, test results, or concerns, I grew more dependent on myself and no one else.

Cancer offers a life that begins with your toes curled over the edge of a cliff, staring into the unknown. But, as you step away from the edge and toward a life of healing and survivorship, you gain a new perspective and way of living. It doesn't happen overnight. But, as you survive each day, you learn to negotiate this new lifestyle. Day in and day out, you ebb and flow, realizing your unwelcome visitor is here to stay. You must recognize that this new version of your life can and will contain hope and promise.

What does this new life offer? The obvious—an appreciation that life changes instantly—and the not-so-obvious: that life will make you stronger in all its glorious mess. Here are my suggestions for finding your new horizon after a cancer diagnosis. It begins with turning toward the complex nature of your situation and facing it head-on. It's a new life waiting for you—embrace it. It's the only one you've got.

Acceptance and Amor Fati

If a superpower existed to help mothers on their cancer journey, I would want it to be the ability to accept everything. Accepting cancer as your new normal is complex, and making peace with your fate takes time. Eighteen years after my diagnosis, I still struggle to accept what has befallen me. I fought against my reality for years—crying, complaining, feeling sorry for myself, being angry—all warranted, but ultimately, it got me nowhere. Wasting time fighting the truth of my situation was exactly that, a waste of time. Only when you accept your diagnosis, the treatments, and the impact on your family can you begin to find stability and peace in your journey.

What are the "dos and don'ts" of finding acceptance? It takes more than simply repeating to yourself, *I accept my reality: I have cancer*. While acknowledging it is a commendable first step, fully embracing something that threatens to destroy your life is incredibly difficult.

To start, consider gratitude. Frankly, I've never been good with gratitude. The word and concept have become understandably ubiquitous in our culture. Some days, I feel like a gratitude flunky because I'm not constantly feeling it, speaking it, journaling about it, and living it all at once. Admitting this seems almost tone-deaf. I can hear the chorus of healthy people saying, "Geez, lady, you've outlived your initial prognosis, your cancer treatment is just a daily pill, and you have a problem with gratitude?" Yes, the fact that I live to see each day gives me reason enough to be grateful.

My challenge comes in the inner conflict of loving my life and all its mess with opposing feelings of anger over my health and jealousy of healthy people—it's a love-hate relationship. Am I grateful for the life-saving medicine that keeps my leukemia in remission and the doctors and researchers who developed this groundbreaking treatment? Yes. Am I thankful for the health insurance that covers the astronomical costs of my care and the ability to see the best oncologists for my disease? Without question. As a mother, I am grateful for innumerable things—just hearing my children fight or listening to some drawn-out story of teen angst means I am here and alive.

But invariably, my mind drifts to those who are not so lucky, to the mothers who did not make it. I have followed many of their courageous stories online and cried for their children. Am I thankful I didn't have *their* cancer? Am I grateful my treatment doesn't include surgery or more aggressive chemotherapy? That feels selfish and confusing. And just like that, my gratitude practice flies out the window in a flurry of doubt.

And then I discovered *amor fati*, the Latin term for loving your fate. Before you judge and call me crazy, stay with me here. The controversial German philosopher Friedrich Nietzsche described his idea for human greatness as amor fati—a love of fate: *"That one wants nothing to be different, not forward, not backward, not in all eternity. Not merely bear what is necessary, still less conceal it . . . but love it."*[4]

Love cancer? No thanks.

But Nietzsche continues, *"Treating each and every moment—no matter how challenging—as something to be embraced, not avoided. To not only be OK with it, but love it and be better for it. So like oxygen to a fire, obstacles and adversity become fuel for your strength. The goal is not 'I'm OK with this.' Not, 'I think I feel good about this.' But, 'I feel great about it. Because if it happened, then it was meant to happen, and I am glad that it did when it did. I am going to make the best of it.' If the event must occur, respond with amor fati. Yes, it's a little unnatural to love things we never wanted to happen in the first place. But what other, worse adversities might this one be saving us from? What might we learn from this unchosen experience? What good, equally unexpected events might result from it."*[5]

I've experienced countless unexpected and positive events in my life because of cancer. I bet you have too. Now, I don't love a disease that could potentially kill me. But, the part of amor fati that believes maybe my cancer was meant to happen resonates with me. You may wonder, *What did I do to deserve cancer?* The truth is, you didn't do anything to deserve it. Yet, here you are. The cards didn't fall in our favor. Even so, we must recognize that we cannot change fate, so we must shift our mindset and ask: What can I embrace and learn from it? And most importantly, how can I model behavior with my family that leaves a favorable impression of who I am and how I faced this adversity?

Amor fati doesn't mean you have to love cancer. Frankly, I hate everything about it. I yell, scream, and occasionally throw horrific tantrums over the inequity of my situation. However, I work hard to accept my leukemia and amor fati the hell out of my life. I choose to embrace strength in the face of adversity, acceptance—but not inaction—and understanding above all else. The good will not always outweigh the bad. Still, embrace all of it. And here's the irony: maybe you'll be grateful for amor fati.

I know this all seems oversimplified. Cancer is complicated. I understand your journey might feel like a living nightmare from which you think you will never wake up. You owe it to yourself not to contemplate all you believe you have lost but to think about what you might gain. It's a mental paradigm shift to love your fate.

I remember the transformative moment when this happened. A few weeks after my CML diagnosis, a fellow mother called to ask how I was doing. As I stared at my floor strewn with my children's toys, the dishes in the sink, and a mound of clean laundry sitting in the basket, the words tumbled out of my mouth, "I am so lucky." Out of nowhere, it all clicked. It struck me that I *do* get to live this life. I'm married, have three beautiful daughters, and I get to be their mom. Yes, I've cried buckets over the cards I've been dealt, but they are mine, so I choose to play my hand.

The Dos and Don'ts of Accepting Your Journey

This list is born out of my mistakes by *not* doing what I preach. I hope you'll find those that work for you and put them into practice. Are these tips obvious? Yes. Difficult? Of course. But maybe my failure to do these things will be your gain.

- ✓ **Don't think about where you are today; do think about where you might be tomorrow.**

Throwing up after an arduous course of chemotherapy makes it hard to think about tomorrow, let alone the next five minutes. As you progress through treatments, fixate on feeling better in the moment. Because that moment leads to another, and then another, until the day is finished—not wasted, not lost, and perhaps not spent with your children, but a day completed. String together enough days, and you have a week. Cross off the hours, days, and weeks you need to endure the most challenging parts of your treatment.

Instead of dwelling on what I missed on a lousy day with cancer and envying others who got to be with my kids while I lay in bed, I focused on what I had completed. I learned to focus not on getting weaker but on how I was improving. My medication became a necessary evil to endure. I had to suffer feeling shitty on one day to make it to the next. It's so much easier said than done, I know. Treatment side effects can set you back mentally and physically for days, weeks, or even months. However, when conditioned to tap into it, there is a reservoir of strength in all of us that can mobilize you, in even the smallest ways, to move forward. And moving forward, whether mentally or physically, is the key to mastering cancer and focusing on your new horizon.

✓ **Don't think you might not live to see your children grow up; do enjoy your time with them now.**

If I could reclaim the countless hours I spent searching the internet for treatment options, statistics, clinical studies, and trials—anything to give me hope—I would. I convinced myself that if I could find the magic bullet that would result in a cure, I would live to see my daughters grow up. And do you know what happened? I missed the very thing I tried to accomplish. I struggle to remember months, if not years, of my children's lives. I was often tuned out to them and into my cancer. This constant worry about my health diverted my attention away from my girls.

Tune into your children as much as you're able. Notice what they do and become aware of their feelings. Sure, you will screw up and lose it when you feel awful. There will be days when, even though you should be celebrating your child's good grade, a school award, or other achievement, you feel depressed. On days like these, allow cancer to do the one thing it's good at: make you more mindful of the passage of time. You might not drop everything to meet your child's every whim, but listen more closely, watch with intention, and love with abandon. If you already do this, high-five for you. If not, extend yourself grace, regroup and pay attention now.

✓ **Don't think about death; do think about living.**

You might be thinking, *Death? Who told me I'm going to die?* No one. But it can be hard not to think about death when you have cancer. No matter how often my oncologists told me I would likely have a good outcome, I saw their eyes. There were no promises. Don't beat yourself up if you, too, think about dying—you're human. When thoughts of death overwhelmed me, I forced myself, with the help of my therapist, to put them where they belonged: in time-out. Like disciplining an errant child, I would repeatedly tell myself, *I don't need to think about this right now,* and did my best to put the thoughts aside. Sometimes I succeeded; sometimes I didn't. Remember, there will always be a time and place to process these feelings—with your therapist, in a support group, by journaling, or speaking with your oncologist, but outside of that—*live.*

- ✓ **Don't let your limitations limit you; do find ways to adjust your lifestyle.**

I bring a worn blue duffle bag with me each time I travel. This ugly bag has frayed edges and looks like it holds sports equipment. Far from it, this duffle contains a machine I use daily to clear my chest of the sticky mucus that cystic fibrosis creates. This mucus can clog my lungs and make me sick. If I don't do the treatments, my lungs feel heavier and dragged down by—for lack of a medical term—crap. In addition to using the machine every day at home to improve my lung function, I bring it with me every time I travel. Additionally, I consume, or inhale, at least five medicines daily for leukemia and CF, seven days a week, 365 days a year. No breaks. Some days, the whole situation frankly pisses me off. But considering the alternative, I adjust my attitude. Eighteen years later, I accept it as part of who I am.

Are there elements of your cancer that limit you? Are you afflicted with side effects of your treatment that affect what you can and cannot do physically? Can you adjust your lifestyle around them? Does your chemo prevent you from doing something you once did with joy? Don't let it go—screw cancer and find a way to do it differently. And then, do it that way repeatedly, so it becomes your new norm. Can't run five, ten, or twenty miles a week any longer? Walk two or even one. Cancer sometimes forces us to change what we love, causing great disappointment. And this includes being a parent.

Maybe the exhaustion of caring for yourself and your family depletes you. Adjust your lifestyle so you can be a mom to your kids, even if it means doing things you found unacceptable before. Accept your limitations and adjust. I let my daughters watch more Disney movies than I care to admit, but I watched with them. I sometimes felt guilty as I lay on the couch with them, feeling awful, but at least I could hold their hands while doing it. Dragging a lung machine on a family vacation isn't fun, nor is inhaling three medications and popping pills in public, but I don't care. And neither should you. Find ways to adjust your lifestyle to fit your new—hopefully temporary—life with cancer. Lose the sadness, frustration, and guilt; they benefit no one. Take immediate action to make your new life with cancer, restrictions and all, work for you and your family.

✓ **Don't push yourself past a healthy point; do recognize you are sick.**

Motherhood can be exhilarating and exhausting, sometimes all at once. There are days you love it and an equal number of days when you don't exactly like your children needing you 24/7. You need a break, especially when you have cancer. Hopefully, your spouse or partner will be there to pick up the slack. But sometimes you might be forced to parent even when you're least able. This is what makes cancer and motherhood so frustrating. You want to do everything the way you did before. You were able to handle adversity, right? But with cancer, everything becomes amplified, more complex, and harder to manage.

In these moments, it's essential to recognize your limits and seek support wherever you can. Remember, you're fighting a formidable opponent. You don't have to be everything to everyone all the time. Know that even in the toughest times, you're doing your best—and that's enough. Know when to pause and set boundaries on your path to recovery. It will be frustrating—nobody likes feeling like the "sick mom." But acceptance is key. Yes, you may be the sick mom with cancer now, but it won't be that way forever, just for now.

If the preceding list feels like it boils down to a Nike *Just Do It* advertisement, that's my intention. Care for yourself first and foremost, and accept what you can and cannot do. Acceptance empowers you to advocate for what you need and then move forward slowly, doing what you can when you can and nothing more. I cannot stress this enough—we start our journey to healing only once we accept that our fate is temporary, not forever.

KEY REFLECTIONS

Accepting what life gives or forces upon us requires opening up to the possibility of living (and loving) a life we never imagined for ourselves. It takes grace and strength to make this adjustment—grabbing hold of what we can have while letting go of what we had envisioned for ourselves. But, our fate holds more than painful cancer moments, especially when we realize that we can accept our reality moment by moment, bit by bit, until our reality becomes something that we feel thankful to have. *Amor fati* and play the cards you hold.

5

When the Cavalry Leaves

The Early Steps to Self-Sufficiency

Soon after your diagnosis, everyone you know and some you don't expect come out of the woodwork. Friends, neighbors, colleagues, and even strangers will hear your story and show up to provide love and support. And food. Lots of food. Or maybe you decided not to tell anyone about your cancer. Your spouse or family members have been assisting you, but no one else. All become your saviors. But, as time passes, people return to their everyday lives, and the web of people who propped you up move on. They aren't insensitive; they're human. Naturally, the people who supported you initially fade away. As they say, the cavalry leaves. At first, this process feels a little scary. Then, slowly, you take your first steps toward self-sufficiency in managing your disease. You feel frightened but also empowered.

Weeks after everyone who came to help after my diagnosis had left, I stood over the kitchen sink, peeling an orange, staring aimlessly out the window. I had momentarily stepped away from my laptop, where I spent an abnormal amount of time relentlessly scrolling for clues that I would survive leukemia and live to see my children grow up. Alex had returned to work, and my girls resumed their regular school schedules. Everyone had restarted their lives — everyone but me.

In the abnormal quiet, left alone with my depressing thoughts, I fixated on the trees swaying in the wind and the azaleas blooming under the bright spring sky. Alternately mesmerized by the swaying branches and the explosion of color in our garden, I lost track of time as I tried to rest my anxious mind. Casually, I glanced at my watch. It was 2:15. 2:15?! Crap, I was late.

Panicking, I remembered it was my turn to drive the afternoon carpool. Six children, including my three girls and some neighborhood kids, would be waiting for me in front of the school. After relying on others to shuttle my girls to and from school and activities, my turn to repay their countless favors had arrived. I had exhausted my last-minute requests for people to help me; I couldn't escape it. I pictured the smiles on my girls' faces as they saw me pull up in front of the school. I couldn't be late. For once, it would be me picking them up, not another parent. Seeing me, I knew they would expound on all the details of their day. There would be discussions about what they ate for lunch and whom they sat with. Perhaps they had a bad day and needed to share that instead. Thinking of this as I scrambled to find my keys brought me a surprising sense of joy. Carpool used to feel like one of those obligatory parental responsibilities you didn't hate but didn't love either. Now, it seemed extraordinarily wonderful — a task I could do to avoid my doom-filled thoughts. I caught myself thinking, "I can't have cancer, I have carpool!"

What once felt like a mundane task I did for the family suddenly gave me hope. And while driving carpool had been a regular part of my life for years, at that moment, for some inexplicable reason, it became my purpose. My health might have been swirling out of control with no guarantee of what might happen, but there was one thing I could do and do well—take care of my children. I could help myself by helping others—namely my family. I realized that motherhood, with all its demands and requirements, would be a life raft in cancer's uncertain waters.

I grabbed my keys.

Looking back, I realize the emotions surrounding my cancer drove my reaction to nearly everything. Doom, gloom, fears, and tears combined to distract me from life and render me paralyzed until I realized motherhood could help combat it. Taking control as a mother helped me feel empowered and in control of my life. I felt empowered to use my parenting responsibilities to help deflect emotions and build a sense of self-sufficiency. You see, with cancer, fear takes on many forms for you, your family, and your friends. So, everyone wants to help and be supportive in the early days following a diagnosis. They fear and hope for the same outcomes you do. But, when the cavalry leaves and returns to their lives, you must fend for yourself. This truth isn't a poor reflection of anyone in your inner circle; it reflects reality. I learned to accept help from the countless people who stepped up to assist our family early on. But, as time passed, I knew it would all come down to me.

By promoting self-sufficiency, I am not condoning selfish, inwardly directed behavior. Shutting everyone out to bolster yourself will not serve you. Self-sufficiency requires a delicate balance of letting love and help in when you genuinely need it while developing your inner mantra of *I'll take it from here* if all else fails.

Ultimately, I knew everything about my health would be up to me. Even my husband could not attend every doctor's appointment or clinic visit because of his responsibility to support our family. So, I figured it out. From that day in my kitchen, I walked my way to self-sufficiency one step at a time. Self-sufficiency and a sense of control felt within my reach; I just needed to find them. And so can you.

EARLY STEPS TO SELF-SUFFICIENCY

My doctors often describe me as a force to be reckoned with. They consider me a Type A personality, armed with too much information and too many questions—not necessarily the most flattering description, but I accept it. I haven't always been this way. My personality has been honed after years of caring for myself. But I know who I am and what I need after years of battling cancer.

Understanding what type of person you are and clarifying what you need to feel in control of your situation is imperative. Do you prefer an all-guns-blazing method to tackle your health or a calm, methodical approach that doesn't leave you rattled after each doctor's visit or treatment? Do you want psychological support, or can you go it alone? Do you want to manage your cancer daily or only face it when you have to? There is no right or wrong way to become self-sufficient. Figure out what works for you.

For example, I discovered the best way to prevent my life from lurching from side to side with each medical encounter was to adopt a systematic and informed approach to my health. As I've stated before, I believe information is power, so I scour the internet for the latest data on my disease. I research all aspects of my illness and then choose what I can apply to make me feel more confident about what will and will not work in my life, especially as a mother.

A cancer-busting diet, for example, would have been great to adopt, but I found it too challenging to execute with small children. Preparing special meals for myself and then different food for my family proved too demanding, requiring extra time and energy I did not have. Cookbooks and printouts of recipes for cancer survivors lined my shelves and lived alongside stray toys and school memos. Ultimately, however, my three small daughters vied for my attention every day. Poring over recipes with hard-to-shop-for ingredients fell to the bottom of my priority list. I wanted to spend more time on the playground and less time cooking over a stove. Every day was precious. Realizing this, I ditched cooking-for-cancer methods and instead tried to eat as healthy as possible. If I slipped, so be it. I wanted to focus on other areas and align those with my day-to-day health. Many of you, however, will smartly focus on diet to beat your disease. I applaud you—you're taking control and doing all you can to beat cancer.

Whatever methods you employ to manage the stress surrounding your disease, do it every day if you can, without fail. For example, different forms of exercise became critical for me. The numerous medicines I consumed fatigued me, so movement helped combat this drag on my body. I scheduled my day to include exercise and other activities for myself and then added in my children's demands to ensure it all got done. Essentially, it became mornings for me to focus on my health and afternoons for the kids. Not much different than before cancer, but somehow, it seemed different. I felt more in control and could better focus on my children once I devoted time to my health, both physically and mentally.

I learned this lesson: if you find a method, process, or activity that supports you and your health and helps you feel empowered, do it. Find what works and master these areas. You can do this—just keep putting one self-sufficient foot in front of the other. Life might go on for those around you, but when you take control and move in the right direction, your life moves forward too.

Consider these other ideas on how to build your self-sufficiency:

✓ Trust Yourself and Your Doctors

Self-sufficiency requires a lot of "trusts." The first thing I learned to trust was myself and my instincts regarding what worked for me in my cancer journey. This trust in myself helped me feel secure in making decisions about my health. I also knew I had to trust my doctors, so I worked to foster a strong relationship with each of them. Together, we formed a working arrangement with rigorous attention to detail and information to formulate my care decisions. It wasn't always easy. Oncologists come in many shapes and sizes—some with egos, some without. I sought ways to find a common bond through shared interests by discussing our kids or sports, for example. This familiarity broke down impersonal barriers so that they felt a connection with me, or so I hoped. I worked hard to build a rapport that would keep the quality of my healthcare high and my doctors' interactions with me at their peak. I found oncologists who would treat my heart and soul as much as the cancer in my body.

I also learned that if I didn't trust—let alone like—one of my attending physicians, I moved on. Fortunately, I haven't had to do this often, but if a doctor ever demeaned me or seemed put off by my countless questions, I found someone else. My life was too short to waste on an uncomfortable doctor-patient relationship.

✓ Trust Science

In addition to trusting myself and my doctors, I had to trust science. Every day I pumped my body with chemotherapy medicine that made me feel ill. But, if I wanted to live to see my daughters grow up, I needed to trust what my oncologists prescribed from day one. I believed in their knowledge, understanding, and familiarity with the science behind my treatment plan.

Yet I also did my research, and so should you. I taught myself to read clinical studies like an expert. Educating myself on my medication and the research to support it informed me of what I could expect—both the good and the bad. I also followed CML survivors well-versed in all aspects of our shared disease on the internet. Seek out these individuals in chat rooms and blogs to answer your questions about your treatment regimen, medications, and clinical trials to understand everything about the science of your cancer. You can spot these patient experts on the internet because they distill important facts into digestible information and point you to clinical studies to read, leading oncologists and specialists to follow, and health advice to adhere to, all while doling out encouragement and empathy in equal measure. I asked countless questions and for guidance, no matter how uninformed I appeared. I didn't care, nor did they. My life was on the line.

Over time, I grew confident enough to comment in online leukemia chat rooms when a new patient would post a question about drug side effects or feelings about their situation. It felt so empowering to offer advice or information to a CML newbie. I attended oncology conferences while working for a cancer nonprofit to hear the leading CML researchers worldwide present their latest research. My ultimate badge of honor came years after my diagnosis when my oncologist quipped after a routine check-up that he wished his research fellows knew as much as I did about CML. While joking, I took very seriously how far I had come in educating myself on the science of my disease. I learned to trust science because I knew science would save me. That fueled my hope and feeling of being in control—an A+ way to promote self-sufficiency.

✓ **Choose Your Tribe to Survive**

Some call the people who support them on their cancer journey their tribe, wolf pack, or circle of support. Whatever you call it and whoever you turn to, identify the cadre of people who truly understand you. These individuals who know you inside and out will tolerate a rant, a cry, a request to listen, or a crazy ask to do something that will make you feel better. Identifying these people, however, might be harder than you think.

Weeks after arriving home from the hospital, my cousin came to town to help with our children. Still reeling from my new reality, I felt grateful for her presence and helping hands. Calm and steady, she did whatever we needed. Like everyone in my life, I could tell she tried hard to contain her shock over the situation Alex and I now faced. But if my cousin felt scared for us, she never showed it. No stranger to chronic illness, my cousin had courageously battled clinical depression for years and had wandered through her own medical maze in search of the best treatment.

One morning, we sat in the kitchen talking after the kids had left for school. I asked if she could impart any wisdom on navigating my new life with chronic disease—something I could latch onto to give me perspective. Although cancer and clinical depression are nothing alike, I felt desperate for any advice from someone who had experience with a long-term illness.

She paused while considering her answer and then shared: "Eat three square meals a day."

Eat three meals a day? I asked myself, wondering if I had heard her correctly. I faced life-threatening leukemia and another disease that would cause my lungs to grow weaker by the year, and I needed to focus on breakfast, lunch, and dinner? My cousin's advice did not mean eating organic, macrobiotic, or cancer-fighting nutrients. Instead, she suggested a general food-balanced approach to feeling better.

Immediately, I knew I had made an error. I learned my first lesson in carefully considering whom to turn to for advice or understanding. While my cousin offered her guidance with loving compassion, I realized it fell short of what I needed. This was not a criticism of her but a wide-eyed critique of myself. She genuinely wanted to impart wisdom she believed might help. But I knew—I needed a different Tribe.

Prudent advice like eating three square meals a day might have been helpful if that was what I needed, but it wasn't. Before asking my cousin, I should have carefully considered the information or advice I sought first and who could best provide that to me. Outside of medical questions, which only my medical team could answer, I wanted people who knew me well enough to offer advice or opinions sympathetically, straight up, or have the courage to say they don't know—no easy task.

Equally, if I need someone who will listen to me rant or vent about my situation, I want them to do just that—listen. One of my dear friends, a master listener, always starts with an empathetic nod and a simple "mm-hmm." Then, after I've finished and she's had a moment to think, she shares her thoughts, or not. Exactly what I need, but that's what works for me. What do you need from your Tribe?

Your Tribe can be as big or small as you like, as many as two or twenty people. Make sure you can trust these individuals with the details of your disease; they understand your emotions and are nonjudgmental. It's about quality, not quantity. Pick and choose those who will serve your best interests—people who really know you. Trust me, it's more complicated than you think.

Only one family member has been in my Tribe from the beginning—my husband. But even that comes with its challenges. Yes, he's my rock and North Star, yet he also has to live with me. And that's the difference. Many in your support network will listen intently, absorb information, offer advice, and then bow out. They don't have to live with your cancer 24/7. A spouse, partner, or close family member doesn't have that luxury. They are always around and, therefore, regularly experience the highs and lows of your journey. Like the rollercoaster you are on, they never get off the ride with you. Living with someone with cancer can be tiring, no matter your level of self-sufficiency and how much you manage your disease on your own. But, just as you never get to put your disease aside, neither do they.

Your doctor(s) should be part of your Tribe. Sadly, for many, their doctor is just the clinical person standing before them, sharing test results and discussing the next steps. Early on, I realized that I needed more from my cadre of doctors and wanted them in my Tribe. I suffered not just physically but emotionally. Like you, I sometimes broke down and cried before my care team. I would've seriously suffered without a friendship backing up our clinical interaction. I needed a casual as well as professional approach to my care. That way, they knew me as more than just a patient when discussing serious issues.

These select family members, friends, and doctors in my Tribe reminded me that I was never alone. Despite my best efforts to subconsciously run them off when I felt down and threw myself a pity party ("I don't need anyone! I can manage this cancer all by myself!"), they ceaselessly had my best interests at heart. And, through thick and thin, they remained by my side. They gave me strength, instruction, and support when I needed it the most. But in the end, as always, I had to be self-sufficient. Lean into your Tribe for support, but also build your self-sufficiency, as you may often find yourself alone on your journey with cancer.

✓ **Know Who Should NOT Be in Your Tribe**

Just as you know the people who should be in your Tribe, you will also know who should not be. I don't need to elaborate here—trust your instinct. Even if someone is your best friend, sister, or brother, they might not provide the consistent, reliable support you need. Perhaps they have too many opinions on how to manage your health or think they have the perfect advice to make you feel better. Except, you never wanted their opinion or their advice. Maybe you just wanted them to listen. Again, it's not their fault. It's your responsibility to identify the right people.

The most crucial part of forming your Tribe is that no matter what happens, if a family member or friend walks away or says something insensitive, you are strong enough to let them go. Once more, self-sufficiency will have taught you to rely on yourself first.

✓ **Keep On Keeping On with Your Friends**

As a cancer patient, only you can decide what you need and what you don't need in your life. Take some time to reflect and identify which non-Tribe friends have been genuinely supportive in the ways that mattered most to you. I discovered over time that these were the ones who were never afraid to ask, "How's it going?" or "How are you?"—and we both knew what they really meant.

I love these people because, while they weren't suitable for my Tribe, I always felt safe sharing an update or two. If someone cared enough to ask, whether a neighbor or a work colleague, even if they risked hearing a lot from me, I considered them worth staying in contact with. At a minimum, I made a point to say hello or ask about *their* lives because they had so gently inquired about mine. And we all know talking about someone else's problems sometimes feels infinitely better than talking about your own.

Unfortunately, some friends and colleagues might drift away during your cancer journey. They might feel uncomfortable with your illness or be afraid to ask how you're doing—some folks can't handle cancer. Ultimately, you get to decide if you want to reestablish the friendship and what you want from it. Maybe you want to share it all—the good, the bad, and the ugly—and you need someone who can handle the spectrum. Or maybe you'd prefer not to talk about cancer at all. Tell folks that; trust me, they will be relieved they don't have to dance around an uncomfortable topic. Bottom line, you get to define the boundaries when you remain friends with certain people or reconnect with those who drifted away.

✓ **Foster Non-Cancer Friendships and Connections**

Take time to connect with people who may not know about your disease. Religious groups, professional or volunteer organizations, or other hobbies offer interaction with people who don't know you have cancer. What about that woman at work who you always wanted to be your mentor? Reach out and form a bond that focuses on your career, not your disease. Isn't that refreshing? Or maybe the time has come to finally take that art class you've been interested in. Feeling like a member of any group will boost your morale.

Want to know the best part? You get to decide if you even want to talk about cancer. There may be certain people you missed seeing because they made you laugh, but they don't have the slightest idea about your latest round of chemotherapy. That's OK! If they made you feel good, and you miss them—reach out, grab a drink, and reconnect. Leave your disease at home. These connections are meaningful because they help you feel true to yourself, capable, and independent. Take that, cancer.

KEY REFLECTIONS

Cancer happens to you first. Then, it ripples through the concentric circles of people in your life, starting with your immediate family. How you interact and communicate with these people will, in many ways, determine the tone of your journey. It is not uncommon for people to fade into the backdrop, but they want to help. They care; they just get lost in their own responsibilities and forget that you still need them.

Take responsibility for developing your self-sufficiency, advocate for your health, outline what you need, and frankly, pursue it. Your friends and loved ones want to help. And perhaps, when all the immediate noise subsides, that is precisely when you need them the most.

6

The Ultimate Conflict

Caring for Yourself While Caring for Your Family

Cancer injects numerous unexpected and unwelcome conflicts into your life. As you move from diagnosis to treatment, recovery, and survivorship, you navigate a never-ending path full of twists and turns that demand your attention and focus. This unwanted journey siphons time away from your family and the version of your life you desperately want back. You want to be present for the world around you, but you feel like crap. You want to remain a strong, capable, and engaged mother, but cancer leaves you feeling exhausted and lacking energy. And we all know children require a lot of energy. You want to interact with your kids as you once did. But cancer comes along and says, *Stop right there, sister.*

Most mothers find that navigating their health while trying to raise their family poses the ultimate conflict when fighting cancer. This aspect of their disease feels the saddest—losing precious time with their children to care for themselves. Even as you become more self-sufficient and start to feel stronger and more confident physically, your outward display of strength may not reflect how you feel inside; you might feel weaker emotionally. Part of your self-sufficiency must involve taking time for yourself—a lot of time.

How do you perfect the art of caring for yourself while also caring for your family? How do you prioritize yourself as the most important person right now, instead of your children? Many might argue that children shouldn't be the sole focus of a mother's life, and I agree. Carving out time for myself has never been a problem; I believe in Me Time as much as you probably do. But now, negotiating what you used to call Me Time—a night out with your girlfriends, a solo walk or run, a quiet bath—feels like Cancer Time. It's an ongoing effort to find pockets of solitude to lie down or catch your breath. What used to be time for yourself is now needed to recuperate from the latest round of chemo, radiation, or other treatments, which, of course, is no fun.

BALANCING SELF-CARE AND FAMILY CARE

Give Up Control

Caring for yourself requires strength and resolve. But sometimes, part of being strong is knowing when you are not. "But wait," you say, "you told me to be self-sufficient! You told me no one will take care of me as well as myself!" While true, self-sufficiency should not and will not prevail *all* the time. It's a fact; cancer will leave you feeling shitty at times. In those moments, I learned and accepted the importance of letting my self-sufficient personality take a back seat.

When you admit weakness, you act more assertively than you think. Acknowledging the need for help and your desire for others to take over requires strength. These moments might be depressing or fuel frustration, but they represent the best care you can give yourself. Let others help you now so you can be better and stronger for your family later. Unfortunately, I learned how to give up control of always managing everything about my health the hard way—by fighting against it.

Sitting on my bed, my hands shook as I prepared an IV infusion of antibiotics to administer to myself. I cried as I squeezed the syringe to inject the medicine into the IV line connected to a port in my arm. Tears of frustration and exhaustion fell onto my lap. I had recently returned home from a lengthy hospital stay for a cystic fibrosis-induced lung infection and felt strung out. Once again, I faced a stint of caring for myself while my husband did his best to maintain a sense of normalcy for our three daughters.

As I sat waiting for the IV to finish dispensing, my husband cautiously entered our bedroom. Alex had learned to dodge my perpetual landmine of emotions carefully. We had argued earlier in the day when he tried to help me with something minor, and I snipped that I could take care of myself. Sadly, self-sufficiency sometimes produces irritable, even irrational, behavior.

Sensing another delicate moment, Alex cautiously asked how I felt and if he could help. I yelled at him again for something stupid, and he understandably hit his own wall of anger. Tired of being my human punching bag and absorbing the blows of my emotional outbursts, he snapped right back at me. As we both dug our feet in the sand, preparing for another battle, I suddenly felt a sharp pain in my chest. My mind raced as I feared an air bubble from the IV had entered my bloodstream. The pain worsened, and I panicked. Sobbing, I shook the syringe and frantically snapped my finger on its side, thinking it would dislodge the imaginary bubbles I thought had entered my vein. Reaching toward me, my husband pleaded to help, but my unreasonable self resisted. "I got it!" I insisted even as my worry grew. As the pain persisted, he suggested we go to the hospital, believing, like me, I might be having a heart attack.

While arguing back and forth, a low but insistent rumbling began outside as an impending thunderstorm approached. I could hear the wind lashing the branches against the side of the house. My chest pain continued, but I didn't waver; I did not want to go to the hospital. I feared the doctors wouldn't release me if I returned. I had just spent an agonizing ten days undergoing rigorous antibiotic treatment to rid me of pesky bacteria affecting my lungs. The emergency room was the last place I wanted to go. Besides, I wondered how we could leave our daughters sleeping in their beds. Do we wake them and explain that Mom has to go to the hospital again? They were just getting used to having me home, no matter my condition.

As the thunder and pelting rain worsened, Alex looked out the window. Then, turning to me, he said sternly, "Beth, we have to go to the hospital. Now." I looked him in the eye and knew—it was time to give up control. My strong personality and self-reliance collapsed in a heap. I yielded to my husband's insistence. Alex guided me downstairs to the car and locked the house behind us. Even as we left our middle school girls at home, we knew they would see our explanation note if they woke up. As we drove through the water flooding the roads, silent relief washed over me that someone had taken over. An hour later, an echocardiogram revealed all was fine—no cardiac arrest. Likely, the liquid medication from my IV had taken a painful route through my bloodstream. My panic certainly didn't help the situation.

Later, I couldn't escape the metaphor of the storm that night. Like Zeus, I tried to command the wind and hold back the tempest. But despite my attempt at being strong in a moment when I felt particularly vulnerable, both physically and emotionally, the storm came. And when it did, I relinquished control and accepted my husband's help. Ultimately, I thanked him for this and, most importantly, the lesson I learned.

Does this experience feel familiar? You may find it natural

to deflect help and strive to be self-sufficient, especially as a woman and a mother trying to embody strength. However, allowing others to help you during inevitable cancer "storms" is essential. I've said it before: sometimes, you must give up control and accept the help you need to get well. Succumbing to others for help does not make you weak.

Extend Yourself Grace

Learning to extend yourself grace when things aren't going your way during your cancer experience—whether you're feeling particularly down, sick, in pain, or didn't receive the test results you hoped for—is crucial. Frankly (and if you're up for it), these can be the best times to be with your family. Turn to your children for distraction, love, or conversation—whatever feels right. Tune out from yourself and into your children. Sometimes, simply being in the same room while each child does their own thing can be all you need.

Here's the truth: I failed at this more often than I succeeded. When my daughters reached middle and high school, I realized almost too late that what mattered most was simply being with them and doing things together. I struggled with the opposite mindset. For years, I talked to my therapist about the same nagging issue—cancer made me feel inadequate, as if I wasn't achieving anything. How absurd is that? Of course, I didn't "achieve" anything; I battled cancer and adult cystic fibrosis every day. But that wasn't good enough for me. I wanted to be a mom, but I also wanted to work. I wanted a career, but I knew working long hours with little time off would harm my health. I felt perpetually frustrated that I couldn't manage it all like many mothers around me appeared to do.

My therapist tried in vain to teach me not to view my life solely as a series of accomplishments. She saw each day as a gift for me, even when I couldn't. She encouraged me to think deeply about what I truly wanted out of life now that I had cancer. Everyone, including my therapist, could easily see that the most cherished things in my life were the eyes of my family staring at me every day.

"Find your bliss," my therapist would say, encouraging me to savor life and seek things that genuinely excited me. The trouble was that I wanted to find my bliss immediately, not while battling cancer. I wanted cancer out of my existence so I could get on with my life as a mother, a wife, a professional—a healthy, whole person. Instead, cancer kept pulling me down to a place of depression, frustration, and the unending, what ifs? *What if I die? What if I never get to live my dreams? What if someone else raises my children? What if, what if, what if.*

"Take a year," my therapist would continue in our sessions, "and figure out what makes you happy outside of cancer. Take the time to figure out what you want to do next," she tried on and on. But time is a precious commodity when you have cancer; you can practically feel the disease pulling you back when you only want to move past it. Each time I tried to heed my therapist's advice, I got edgy and impatient rather than taking the time needed to understand my identity outside of cancer and what I wanted from life. Instead, I would jump at professional freelance projects or part-time assignments. Quickly cycling through what I thought I wanted felt easier than sitting quietly with myself and appreciating being alive and with my kids. Leukemia had a way of playing with my mind just enough to keep me perpetually busy so I wouldn't hear the "what ifs" swirling in my head.

Looking back, I wish I'd been more judicious in my choices—overtiring myself with "doing things" left me with less energy for my kids. I grew grumpy as I battled fatigue from my treatment, mothering, and random professional assignments. Perpetually trying to prevent cancer from holding me back, I exhausted myself by competing with no one but my ego. *Cancer doesn't have a hold on me,* I told myself, *I decide my life.* Yes, I did decide my life, but cancer became the driver.

Don't make this mistake. Know where to draw the line. Let cancer be your teacher, not your competitor. Care for yourself and your family first. Extend yourself grace; don't allow cancer to compel you to prove who's boss. We know you're the badass of your life, not cancer.

Getting Help to Help Yourself

We've discussed previously how self-sufficiency often means getting help to help yourself. Learn to work together with your family, friends, doctors, and care team to operate at peak performance with your limited energy. Don't allow pride to keep you from asking for assistance. Sometimes, our foolish, sabotaging beliefs make us afraid of appearing weak. Mothers may excel at many things, but we all have our vulnerabilities, especially when facing cancer. And without a helping hand, we will not thrive. So, ask yourself, "What do I need, and how can I best get that?"

Below are some of the things I found to be most helpful. You won't need to use all of them at once—just pick and choose what works for you, or create your own approach. Most are abundantly evident, but sometimes, it helps to remind ourselves of the obvious.

- ✓ **Ask Friends or Neighbors to Help with Things They Already Do**

Someone is always going to a grocery store or pharmacy, so if a person asks if they can pick something up for you, you should routinely say yes. And every parent will be happy to swing by your house and grab your child to drive to organized sports or school activities. As you consider the areas where you could use help, why not ask people looking for a way to lend a hand? If a neighbor offers to rake your leaves, let them! It makes them feel good to help, and it's one less thing for you and your family to tackle. A quick interaction when they drop off items or stop by might be just what you need—short and sweet. Don't feel obligated to discuss your feelings or frustrations, like chemo-induced hair loss. Talk about anything other than cancer. Save those deeper conversations for your closest friends, family, or Tribe.

✓ **Get Help for the Busiest Times of the Day**

When my daughters were little, I hired college girls from four to six p.m. to help with homework, dinner, and the bedtime routine. It maintained my sanity, preserved my energy, and didn't cost a fortune. As they got older, I hired high school girls to pick them up from school and drive them to activities so I could work or rest. Perhaps your older children can help their younger siblings after school. Offer to pay them in whatever currency they prefer: money, a sleepover with friends, or new clothes they may be eyeing. It's worth every penny and will help you immensely.

✓ **Adopt a Lifestyle That Helps You Feel Normal**

Did you attend a book club before cancer? A bible study or other religious group? What about social or professional organizations you were a part of? Did you stop going because of cancer? Then go back. Once you feel stable emotionally and physically, return to the activities you once enjoyed. You may dread the stares, the awkward questions, and the unspoken presence of cancer. But, if you stay home to avoid things because you can't face the music, then cancer wins. Don't let cancer win—ever.

✓ **Pursue Things You Are Interested in or Passionate About**

One benefit of cancer is that it acts as a mirror, reflecting what truly matters to you. As you look into your eyes, ask yourself what you most want right now. Did you hope to volunteer at your children's school but were too busy with work or other commitments? Now is your chance. Are there books you wanted to read but never found the time? Projects you hoped to do with your kids but didn't get around to? Dive into the wonder of things. Learn not to waste one more minute doing something you aren't passionate about. Be sure to temper this, however, with a dose of reality. If you don't have the energy now due to treatment, lack of time, or resources, that's fine. Add them to your list of *Things I'd Love to Do One Day*. This does not constitute a bucket list, a term I despise. Why have a list of things to do before you die (or kick the bucket)? Do you really need the prospect of death to motivate you? I sure don't. My diseases remind me of my mortality every single day. I don't need a list of things to do before I die; I just need a list of things I'd love to do.

My list of *Things I'd Love to Do One Day* remains short and motivating. They become items I can do now (or next week, month, or year). If I encounter or hear about something exciting, it goes on the list, and because I'm interested or passionate about it, I try to make it happen. But, if I never get to it, no problem. Something else, equally interesting, replaces it — no bucket list pressure for me.

✓ **Slow the Hell Down**

Maybe you already do this. Perhaps you've mastered the art of slowing down to focus on daily moments and what holds importance. It's a learned trait for most of us, often challenging without proper focus and reframing. Slowing the pace of your life forces you to prioritize your time and reorient it toward you and your family. For some of you, this will be easy as your disease forces you to spend more time in bed than you care to admit. Slowing down also helps you process your emotions, both the good and the not-so-good, rather than burying them for potential problems later. Don't simply slow down because you've been forced to because of cancer. Get in the habit.

Cancer has handed you a gift you never wanted, but if you allow it, it will repay you with more life lessons than you can imagine. I know you would rather skip the life classes and forget your disease—I get it. But if you learn to treasure the moments when cancer isn't knocking you down, you'll be amazed by the beauty in every little thing around you. Again, I didn't always and still don't always do this. I tried to outrun cancer by staying busy, which at times proved helpful but mostly just wore me out, leaving me a grumpy mom and spouse. Take it from me: slow down and drink in all life offers.

✓ **Simplify Your Life**

Many of us have a way of—well—complicating things. We live lives filled with unnecessary challenges and schedules bursting at the seams. We try to juggle too many things at once, especially as moms. Cancer confronts us enough without all the extra moving parts we add.

If you aim to simplify your life to better care for yourself, start by focusing on what matters most: your health, children, spouse, or partner. Each of these requires plenty of attention. Your children's schedules alone could keep you busy 24/7. Simplifying your life might also mean streamlining your personal responsibilities while continuing to work professionally because work fuels you, or you have to support your family. However you do it, boil everything down to life's essential components and nothing more. Simplifying may seem easy, but executing it, in reality, proves harder.

✓ **Become an Expert Communicator**

Keep your family informed of how you are feeling physically and emotionally. It forms patterns of what they can expect during different times of your treatment. Becoming an expert communicator lets you express your feelings, needs, and wants up front. It might get old having to remind your family each time that, yes, chemo makes you feel like crap. But it pays off.

My oral chemo tired me physically for a few hours immediately after taking it each day. I usually took it soon after my children went to school to recover while they were gone. But on weekends, when everyone was around, I would communicate over and over that I couldn't do much right after taking my medicine. My husband would take over with the kids if I disappeared upstairs after simply stating, "I'm not feeling great." Years later, that's all I have to say, and my husband recognizes my imminent disappearance for a few minutes or hours. I've communicated the same message over the years, so no one is surprised anymore. Now, my family often says they're sorry I don't feel well—they've strengthened their empathy muscles after years of hearing how I am feeling. Sometimes, good can come from bad!

✓ **Find Your Mantra**

A metal plaque on my bedside table reads, *Don't Give Up. Don't Ever Give Up.* If you know the legendary North Carolina State basketball coach Jimmy Valvano, you've probably heard his speech where he echoed a famous Winston Churchill quote. In his 1993 ESPY Courage Award address, given less than two months before his death from adenocarcinoma, Valvano heartfeltly shared, "Cancer can take away all my physical abilities. It cannot touch my mind, it cannot touch my heart, and it cannot touch my soul. And those three things are going to carry on forever."[6]

The motto of his cancer research foundation is *Don't Give Up, Don't Ever Give Up*. So I don't.

Find the phrase, slogan, or image that compels you to keep going whenever you see it. These can be found everywhere: online, in a book, or a photo—choose whatever inspires you. How does this help you care for yourself? Motivational quotes or pictures offer us a quick burst of wisdom to get our focus back, offering the inspiration needed for the day or occasion (blood test, body scan, or oncology appointment). They encourage us when our everyday motivation has lapsed, which unfortunately happens more often than we like.

KEY REFLECTIONS

Challenge yourself to loosen your urge to control each aspect of your life with cancer with an iron grip. You have to give up control and instead give yourself grace. You have to seek help to bring your best self to this battle. Perhaps revealing your vulnerabilities and accepting assistance demonstrate your true strength and wisdom in caring for both you and your family. Actively choosing to fill your life with things that bring comfort and compassion to your days will only make you stronger, allowing you to be the resilient mother and partner you aspire to be.

7

When the Dust Settles

The Infamous "New Normal" Begins

What is normal about cancer? Simply put, nothing. Nothing is normal about something that shatters your life. Yet, weeks, months, or even years after your treatment ends, you will enter survivorship and encounter your "new normal." This phase will likely change your perspective on almost everything. Learning to live as a survivor, navigating your new life, becomes a transformative process that only fellow survivors and members of your Tribe can understand.

Survivorship does bring joy: you have recovered, your family no longer fears your demise, and your future looks bright. The good almost always outweighs the bad. But when the dust settles, your life undergoes a permanent change.

Sitting in the parking lot, consumed with dread, I stared at each person leaving the grocery store, checking to see if I recognized anyone. Silently, I spoke to myself, "You can do this. It's just the grocery store." I looked in the side and rearview mirrors, expecting to see someone walk up to say hello. For weeks, I had been the neighborhood story. Everyone knew the local thirty-eight-year-old mom with twin toddlers and a six-year-old daughter who had recently been diagnosed with a potentially fatal form of leukemia. No one knew I had also been diagnosed with adult cystic fibrosis.

I repeatedly sighed, just wanting to go home and forget the food for my family. They could go hungry. My heart thumped as I debated the pros and cons of grocery shopping—did my kids really need dinner? Ignoring my trepidation, I forced myself out of the car. Entering the store with my head down and face mask secure, I moved expeditiously as I threw items into the cart. I had successfully navigated the produce and bakery aisles without seeing anyone I knew, but when I turned the corner, I came face to face with a neighbor. Spotting me with my mask, which I wore to prevent my leukemia-weakened body from getting sicker, proved easy.

"Oh my gosh, Beth, how arrreee you?" my well-intended neighbor asked as she slowed her cart.

What could I say? Devastated? Heartbroken that I might not live to see my children grow up?

As my neighbor tried not to stare at my mask, I tried acting like the old Beth, casual and easy-breezy, just conversing. I desperately wanted to be my old self, with my old self's minor issues and "problems." But neither one of us bought it. Instead, I stood there attempting to explain how I was doing, and yes, of course, she could bring me a casserole. Numerous shoppers filed by, trying not to look at me—the lady with the mask—but I saw them. When we finished talking, I quickly bought my items and bolted from the store. From that day forward, I realized that most people would know me and my disease. Leukemia brought a new dimension to my life that took time for me to accept, let alone talk about with others. But, whether I liked it or not, I knew this was my new normal.

So many things will be different during and after your cancer journey, whether it's relationships with your family and friends, your work life, or how you live daily. That doesn't mean you can't have healthy and meaningful connections to these changes. Half the battle is overcoming these differences as you move through your journey and enter your new normal.

EXPERIENCING YOUR NEW NORMAL

No two cancer survivors experience their new normal in the same way. Some women will keep working at home or the office while undergoing treatment and continue to do the same in survivorship. They juggle chemo, oncology follow-ups, work meetings, and parent-teacher conferences with composure. Barely skipping a beat, they exude grit and a screw-you-cancer attitude. You go, girl.

For other women, cancer feels like a bomb detonating in their once orderly lives. Suddenly, you become sick, and the emotional shock is almost as great as the physical. Any sense of your former life evaporates, and a new life begins. But not before months of adjusting to treatment and learning to parent children while navigating all the commitments cancer and survivorship demand. It may be new, but it does not feel normal.

I can tell you that what was normal to me as a mother before cancer changed dramatically post-diagnosis. The trivial things immediately fell away. Toys on the floor or a messy home all felt meaningless now that my health and existence were in reasonable question. "Bless this mess" never felt so accurate. The mess felt good, or at least ignorable for once. Who cares if dishes pile up in the sink when you have an upcoming scan or a critical blood test?

What does a load of laundry matter when facing a potential bone marrow biopsy? Of course, I didn't change overnight. It took time to get comfortable with my "messy" new life.

Everyone's new normal is different. Here are some things to consider along the way:

✓ **Spending Your Time Wisely**

Most things do remain normal after a cancer diagnosis. But the priority and attention you give them shifts. Cancer has a way of paring down what truly matters and what does not. I still recall the night I stared at the antiaging cream I routinely applied to my face and wondered, Why bother? How long would I live anyway? Did I need to preserve an outward, youthful appearance? I hyperanalyzed everything that was once a regular part of my life. Is this worth my time? Is that worth my time? Everything felt so tenuous, as if hanging on by a thread.

Of course, everyone must still run necessary errands, go to the dentist, and change the oil in their car: the must-dos of life. What cancer gifts you, however, is clarity, which becomes—or should become—your new normal. How you spend your time crystallizes; you never want to waste it again. Yes, you will devote plenty of time to cancer waiting rooms, chemo chairs, and recovering from treatment. But that is not a waste—it's survival. When you are feeling well again and your life returns to "normal," guard your time and spend it wisely, must-do days and all.

✓ **Being Present vs. Being Productive**

Before leukemia and adult CF, I preferred to "get things done" while my kids attended school, always seeking something that felt productive. As a stay-at-home mom then, I believed it was my responsibility to manage the household and our children's lives. So, I made the most of my time with my children out of the house, or so I thought.

Working out, going to the grocery store, managing the house, and arranging our family's nonstop schedule filled my time. I know you can relate.

In the course of it all, I missed the point. Cancer helped me see what I overlooked. Soon after my life stabilized and I adjusted to treatment, I began observing my life through a changed lens. It's not that I sleepwalked through motherhood before cancer—far from it. Instead, my disease escalated my awareness of the importance of each day. Feeling productive no longer mattered because I realized that simply *living* each day counted as productive. Doing laundry, for example, proved I was still here taking care of my family, and isn't that a gift? Of course, I didn't enjoy washing mounds of clothes for a family of five, but at least *I* did it. What might sound like a New-Agey approach to daily living reflects a simple awareness of your place in life. Doing mundane activities affirmed my life; they did not detract from it.

This awareness also allowed me to view my children's lives differently. I wondered about their day at school, for example. How did they spend their time? Rather than hearing their daily download to the "What did you do in school today?" question, I started volunteering in their classrooms to see for myself. I loved watching my girls' eyes light up when I entered the room. I never missed a sporting event, music or dance recital again. To be clear, I didn't miss many before—but after cancer, I observed different details of these gatherings. I watched the sway of their dresses when they danced; I noticed the wince of disappointment on their faces when they missed a soccer goal or a tennis shot. This clarity, this observation of life—being present and truly seeing it—became my new normal.

✓ **Learning to "Jump the Rails"**

In the months after my diagnosis, people were outrageously kind and generous with gifts, food, and offers to babysit my children. I felt overwhelmed by the prayers, letters, phone calls, and even the kind older man who miraculously appeared at my front door one day with a honey-baked ham. No warning, no phone call—just a retired gentleman who heard about a young mother with cancer in the neighborhood and wanted to help.

But, after a year of abundant attention and love, the pages in the open book of my life began to fray. I no longer wanted everyone to know the status of my cancer and when or if I would get better. I didn't want to share my latest health update or explain how CML works. This experience required a new set of skills to face the world, as I didn't want my disease to be my primary identity.

Slowly, I began to do what I call "jumping the rails" on a fictitious train track in my mind. I adopted this mental concept to feel normal, like an adult version of the children's game Let's Pretend. On one railroad track, I mentally ride the Cancer Train. When I'm on the Cancer Train, I manage my disease with frequent "train stops" at doctor's appointments, daily medications, treatments—you name it, anything associated with my leukemia. This fabricated train runs like clockwork, with medicines taken at the same time each day, regularly scheduled monthly blood checks, and follow-up visits with my doctors. Little change occurs in my schedule on this train—it's what I must do to ensure my disease remains in check. This mental train ride is predictable, and I know what to expect. I force myself, like clockwork, to do what's required to maintain my health.

On the other railroad track in my head, I ride the Normal Train. On this train, I pretend I don't have cancer (this might sound wild and implausible to you, but hear me out). I mentally live the life of other mothers I know—a life without disease and seemingly more carefree. I participate in things where I don't have to talk, let alone think, about leukemia. I joined groups where women didn't know I had two life-threatening diseases.

Inherently, I know that people on my made-up Normal Train have problems too. But on the Normal Train, I can be a passenger free of cancer and adult CF and all the weight that bears. Without my diseases clouding the picture, I can wallow in the same stresses of child-rearing or family issues as other mothers. I can discuss fun topics or ask friends or colleagues about *their* lives. I try to ride the Normal Train in my mind as much as possible. Living without disease offers unique freedom; I don't have this luxury. So, if I occasionally pretend I don't have cancer to feel less weighed down by life mentally, I do it.

"Jumping the rails" is a method I've devised for myself where I can live one life but mentally occupy two worlds. Some would say this is denialism and I'm not being true to myself, that I'm a hypocrite. Many women would argue they don't have the luxury to partake in this mental game because the physical effects of their disease are too great. I understand. But for me, if you walk a mile in my shoes for eighteen minutes, let alone eighteen years, you too would get tired of talking about bombshell diseases like chronic leukemia and adult cystic fibrosis. I've seen too many looks of exasperation and confusion ("She sure doesn't look sick!") on the well-meaning faces of family and friends. Sometimes it's easier to live my life on two different tracks—one where I face my cancer head-on and one where I don't. So I "jump the rails," even if only in my mind. I feel it is my right to choose when I don't want my diseases to be the big, uncomfortable topic. It's not deceitful. It's honest. I'm being true to myself and what I need. It's a new normal for me—living a version of my former life while embracing my new reality.

✓ **Your "Normal" Family Life**

It has been eighteen years since my diagnosis, and happily, my family rarely thinks about my cancer. I go to annual check-ups and blood tests with barely a shoulder shrug from family members when I tell them where I have been. Of course, they ask how the appointment went, but as soon as I answer, they ask some unrelated question: "Glad it went well, Mom. Hey, did you wash my soccer jersey?" What a relief that cancer no longer takes center stage in our lives.

Adjusting to life as a mother with cancer normalizes faster than you think. Family members adapt to your treatment schedule and medical needs out of necessity. Lives must resume their regular pattern for everyone's wellbeing, including yours. You develop a keen appreciation for the consistency school and work provide to maintain a sense of normalcy in your home. Homework, music lessons, sports, or school functions offer a healthy dose of the ordinary. I enjoyed carpooling and orchestrating my children's schedules like never before because they had been, and once again became, a normal part of our lives. That is the goal: achieving a new normal that resembles your family's old normal.

✓ **Friendships: Accepting the Changes**

Part of your new normal involves accepting that cancer will change many things in your life, including friendships. While many changes will be positive, a few might be unwelcome. You quickly learn who feels comfortable with your situation and who does not. I recall one spring afternoon soon after my diagnosis when my husband and I worked outside in our yard. It felt glorious to be outdoors after my hospital stay. As we weeded and planted, a friend barreled up our driveway unannounced, music blaring from his car. He heard through the grapevine that I'd returned home from the hospital and wanted to see me. I stood on our front lawn holding a rake, staring at my friend in disbelief. Who told him I was home? I didn't feel ready to see anyone outside of my family. Sensing my discomfort, my friend rolled down his window and made a humorous comment about my face mask. Admittedly, I did look ridiculous wearing a face mask while raking the yard. But his jokes were just the comedy I needed as he got out of his car to hug me. Humor from friends immediately signals that while they might be uncomfortable with your situation, they strive to put you at ease before themselves. It's a selfless act of love.

Other friends might spare you the exhaustion of answering countless questions about your disease by doing their own research. It's a relief not having to explain your cancer from A to Z in a social situation. These are friends you may grow closer to. At the same time, you might notice some friends spending less time with you, and some friendships might fade completely no matter what you do.

It is essential to understand that cancer will change you too. You might discover a new purpose or become more dedicated to a new cause or hobby. These will lead to new connections and friendships, replacing some you may have lost.

KEY REFLECTIONS

No doubt, cancer disrupts everything normal about your life, from your physical being to your relationships to your activities, schedule, and plans. Adapting to this shift in your life requires you to be flexible in ways that you must embrace, however reluctantly. And, because cancer touches each person in such an individualized way, the "new normal" you take on must be carefully crafted by you. Remembering the essential elements of your life can help you shape the new normal you will live: What do you need? What does your family need? What do you love? What do you value and want to prioritize? As the dust settles, consider this phase of recovery as a new beginning for you to cast aside attitudes and actions that no longer serve you and adopt those that reflect the person you want to be.

8

From Toddlers to Teens to Everything in Between

The Effects of Your Cancer on Your Children

One of the most significant concerns for mothers with cancer involves how it might impact their children. Although kids are often more resilient and less fragile than we think, it's natural to worry about how they will respond to your diagnosis. The severity of the disease, the demands of treatment, and their combined effect on a mother's ability to care for her family all play crucial roles in this concern.

From toddlerhood until my daughters finished high school, my leukemia remained a regular facet of their lives. I spent the first year after diagnosis adjusting to the side effects of my oral medication but seldom found myself bedridden. Various symptoms continued for years, regularly impacting my ability to parent as effectively as I wanted, as CML felt like an unwelcome visitor who never seemed to leave. For other women, however, a cancer diagnosis might resemble a fast-moving storm that blows in, wreaks havoc for a while, and then clears out. It causes intense concern and requires some adjustments, but generally leaves the family unharmed. Cancer never follows a predictable path for any two families.

But what about the effects of your cancer you don't see in your children? The fear or anxiety that your family chooses not to share with you. Or their curiosity about "catching" your cancer. Or even worse, wondering if they caused it in the first place. In the whirlwind of caring for yourself, it can be hard to add another thing to think—let alone worry—about. Through it all, remind yourself that modeling resilience and strength, no matter how positive or negative your experience has been, will be one of the greatest legacies of your experience.

"Mom? What's the name of that medicine you take for your leukemia again?" my twin teenage daughter asked from the living room.

"Gleevec," I replied while putting away groceries and glancing at the television in the kitchen.

"And what year were you diagnosed?" she continued. I could hear her typing on her computer.

"May 6, 2006," I answered, still oblivious to her questions.

"And you take your medicine every day, right?" she continued as she typed. *"Are you in remission?"*

"Yes, and yes," I replied, now curious about her subtle interrogation. I wandered into the living room, holding a head of lettuce. *"Lily, what's with all the questions?"*

"Do you have a picture of yourself I could have?" she asked, ignoring me as she continued to type.

"Lily, what are you doing with all this info?" I asked again.

"I'm starting a fundraiser with my friends for the Leukemia and Lymphoma Society (LLS). We're trying to raise the most money, and if we do, we get the 'Fundraiser of the Year' award

and a cash prize. It's so cool. We're raising the money in your honor," she continued typing furiously. "I'm drafting an email to my friends and setting up our fundraising page."

It had been fifteen years since my diagnosis. Just two years old at the time, Lily was too young to remember the mayhem my cancer caused. Thankfully, I had been in deep remission for much of her teenage years, so neither she nor her sisters inquired about my disease. Aside from my parents, no one asked anymore, and I rarely spoke of it.

"Uh, Lily, wait. I'm not sure I want to be a cancer poster child again," digesting what my daughter told me.

Although my husband had raised thousands of dollars and widely shared my story during my first year with leukemia, my cancer was no longer the talk of the neighborhood.

"Lily, stop typing for a minute and look at me. Why are you sending this?" I asked, not wanting to relive my story with my daughter's friends and complete strangers. The days of sharing details on my health had long passed.

My daughter looked up at me with her fingers poised over the keyboard.

"Mom, what's wrong with it? We're raising money for cancer research. I told you, our team wants to raise $10,000 for the Leukemia and Lymphoma Society," she explained, confused by my reaction.

"I don't know if I want my story out there again, honey. It's been so long," I replied, admiring Lily's determination.

"Why not? Your story is so inspiring, Mom. You're the strongest person I know," she responded, repeating the statement that struck my heart each time I heard it.

For years, my daughters wrote me countless birthday cards and notes that ended with, "You're the strongest person I know." Touched by their words, I felt proud of how I had, for the most part, managed my diseases for so long. Admittedly, however, I sometimes wondered if they wrote it only to make me feel better. I often read their words with a twinge of doubt. "Am I strong?" I would ask. And each time, I reminded myself: Yes, I am. If my children believe I'm strong, then I must believe it too.

I continued staring at my daughter's confused face. "Mom?" Lily asked, "Are you OK?"

"Yes, I'm OK," I said after several moments, returning to the kitchen. "You can send the email."

I heard Lily strike the keyboard, relaying my story once again to hundreds of people I barely knew.

What a revelation: my cancer, diagnosed when Lily was two years old, still resonated with her fifteen years later. My disease had made a lasting impression on my daughter, an indelible imprint she will carry with her forever. And while I thought I had managed my leukemia largely on my own, Lily taught me our children observe and absorb much of what we experience, whether they tell us or not.

HOW YOUR CANCER AFFECTS YOUR CHILDREN: A COMPLICATED PUZZLE

Just as each cancer has its specific makeup and complexity, each family's reaction to a mother's diagnosis and treatment, and the overall impact on home life will be unique. Studies show that over time, children may have a higher risk of emotional and behavioral problems when a parent has cancer. The disruption of schedules and daily routines, shifting of household roles, financial stress, and the lack of physical and emotional availability of either parent contribute to these possible issues. If left untreated or overlooked, the problems could continue into adulthood.[7]

Indeed, your family may also emerge unscathed, but

some areas warrant observation. Understandably, some things I discuss may feel overwhelming or too clinical. This list aims to share the possible effects, both positive and negative, on your children at different life stages. Remember, I believe information is power, so utilize it to your advantage and recognize that not everything will be relevant to you and your children.

✓ **Daily Routine and Emotional Reactions**

We all know children tend to operate best with a daily routine. Despite this, a cancer diagnosis disrupts regular schedules due to mom's frequent oncology and other doctor visits, unexpected hospital admissions, and the home turning into a place of care.[8] According to research, these disruptions may cause preschoolers sleeping problems, increased post-traumatic stress symptoms, and internalizing and externalizing behaviors in teens.

Internalized behaviors are quiet and often invisible because they are generally not disruptive to others. Examples of internalized behaviors in teenagers include anxiety and depression, which can lead to withdrawal from activities and poor academic performance. Externalized behaviors might be apparent and shouldn't be ignored, including being nervous, irritable, withdrawn, eating more or less than usual, feeling afraid or lonely, sad, unloved, or having trouble concentrating.[9] Of course, being a typical high school teenager or a disgruntled middle schooler can also cause many of these problems. It can be hard to ascertain—never hesitate to contact your child's doctor or school counselor if you remain concerned.

Adolescents also report the impact of physical unavailability on their emotional well-being, including the ill mother no longer driving carpool, for example, or attending extracurricular activities.[10] Changes to your household's routine may prove complex for everyone involved. All moms want to stay present in parenting and minimize disruptions to their children's lives due to cancer. By understanding how these changes affect your daily life and the resulting emotional reactions, you can better prepare for the challenges.

✓ **Role Changes**

Role changes between you and your spouse, significant other, or family member may be minor or significant during your cancer. Expect parental role changes as your spouse becomes the caregiver and takes over some of the responsibilities you usually manage. You become less available physically and emotionally during intense treatment periods, having fewer opportunities to interact while placing increased demands on your children. It's understandably hard for all involved.

Research shows that younger children and adolescents may have increased personal responsibilities during these periods, resulting in decreased social activity and subsequent loss of childhood just when peer groups are essential for social development.[11] Your teen, for example, may want to stay home to be with you or help care for their younger siblings. In extreme cases, a teen may pick up extra work shifts to help combat cancer's financial burden on a household.[12] Reassuring your children that these role changes are temporary may help ease their stress and desire to feel that they must "do something" to help out during this challenging time. Encourage them to continue engaging with friends, despite everything happening at home.

✓ **Other Emotions**

Your children may exhibit some of the emotions you experience. Frankly, it's frightening and depressing to think that the emotional toll of your disease could extend beyond yourself. As if being vigilant about your emotional

I Can't Have Cancer, I Have Carpool!

health isn't enough, you must also monitor your children's emotional well-being. There's no question that children coping with a parent's cancer are under tremendous stress. As previously mentioned, they're more likely to experience increases in general levels of distress and anxiety. They may also experience other mood changes that can affect their self-esteem.[13]

The National Cancer Institute reports that young children and teens might also feel guilty. It's important to reassure children in advance, even if they don't express this. You might try a blanket statement such as, "The doctors have told us that no one can cause someone else to get cancer, it's nothing that any of us made happen." [14] Again, do not hesitate to involve a licensed professional for your child to talk to if it is more than you or your family members can handle alone. Consider keeping guidance counselors at school aware of the situation at home so they may work with your teen and their teachers.

✓ **Social Functioning**

A mother's battle with cancer might impact their children's mental health and family cohesiveness. According to Anticancer Research, parents report that frequent appointments and intense treatment plans may increase children's anxiety and depression, which decreases parenting efficiency and, thus, family functioning.[15] They state that preschoolers rely on positive family functioning and exhibit distressed behaviors when their family cohesiveness becomes altered. Elementary school children and adolescents, especially daughters, are affected by their parents' mental state. In response, they learn their own set of coping techniques accordingly. Parents and teachers both report that boys of parents with cancer exhibit more externalizing problems, which further impairs social functioning.[16]

Adolescents report a larger support network, including

friends, counselors, and teachers, than elementary school children. However, they also comment that they sacrificed something fun with friends to stay home due to increased household responsibilities and caretaker roles. For adolescents, providing avenues for them to connect with other peers in similar situations is essential. Teens report better support from friends whose parents also have cancer, as they find it difficult to relate or express ideas to their unaffected friends.[17]

The impact on social functioning with your children is not all negative. Thankfully, there are many opportunities for positive outcomes for your children. As I experienced within my own family, the effect on social functioning with our young daughters was short-lived. As my health stabilized and my cancer became more normalized over the years, our family life morphed back into its pre-cancer routine. As I grew stronger, my girls drifted back to the social patterns they were accustomed to, with fewer diversions needed due to my oncology appointments, clinic visits, and treatment.

Your older children might experience personal growth and thrive despite the challenges and changes they've endured. We've all read incredible stories of teenagers going on to study medicine or other forms of patient care because of their parent's cancer. And, as you read at the beginning of the chapter, they may want to fundraise for your disease. Encourage your adolescents to explore areas they become interested in relating to your condition or survivorship. Perhaps your child helped care for you after treatment or surgery and is now well-suited for nursing. Maybe they become interested in culinary arts because they cooked for you, or they want to dive deeper into areas of holistic care—the options are endless—and hopeful!

- ✓ **Your Children Need You, and You Need Your Children**

   Here's the truth: you need your children during cancer almost as much as they need you. From initial diagnosis to treatment to recovery, your children will likely be around for much of your journey. They need you in their day-to-day lives, and you need them in your recovery to bring you joy and a healthy distraction from cancer.

   Despite this, there will be times when you wish your children would—dare I say it—give you a break. You crave quiet moments to focus solely on yourself and your health. You love being a mom and want your children around, but sometimes the energy required to care for yourself and manage your family feels more than you can bear. Mastering being present and caring for your children while undergoing treatment takes skill. As I mentioned earlier, the easiest place to start is folding them into your life with cancer as seamlessly as possible. Talk openly about what you're experiencing and how it makes you feel. Your children might surprise you with words of empathy or encouragement. Our kids can be our greatest cheerleaders.

   Just as children may cheer you on, they also want to help; supporting their mom might be exactly what they need to feel like they're doing something amid the chaos. Consider asking your children to help around the house. It's a win-win for all involved: less work for you and your children feel they're contributing. But beware of creating unrealistic expectations for assistance. It's about balancing what needs to be done and spending time together doing it versus creating undue stress. No child wants to feel they must do more work because mom is sick. Remember that you cannot expect your children to be expert cleaners or do their chores as carefully as you might. Accepting their best efforts will help keep them motivated;

it's all about balance. Do you honestly care if it is done right or if it just gets done at all?

Consider the following tips when involving your children to help with chores. You might already do some of these things in your home, or they may spark new ideas for you to try. Mothers each have their own parenting style and beliefs, so find your distinct path and guide your family in a way that works for you.

> **Visualize Tasks.** Use a chart to help children and teens keep track of their chores. This chart will clarify your expectations by establishing what tasks need completion and when.
> **Adopt a Team Approach.** Work together to complete larger tasks. For example, to clean up after dinner, you might have one child clear the table and another put away the leftovers.
> **We're All in This Together.** Ask your children to help each other. Younger children can help each other pick up toys or fold laundry. Teenagers and older children can help with car rides and homework.
> **Incentivize!** Build incentives into chores. For example, let your children pick their drink and dessert when they make their school lunch, or heck, don't micromanage it; just let them pack the entire thing with simple guidance.
> **Thank You Goes a Long Way.** Let your child or teen know that you appreciate their help. Say thank you and offer rewards for jobs well done. Rewards may include a family movie night, an ice cream outing, or extra screen time.

KEY REFLECTIONS

Cancer's reach extends past you, your children, and your family. While it's heartbreaking to know that this disease infects not just your body and mind but also the consciousness and behaviors of your kids, you have the opportunity to incorporate them into the healing process in ways that assist all of you. These adjustments provide an opportunity for the strength that you and your children innately have to rise to the occasion as you act in unison to battle and heal from cancer's imposition on your family life.

Ultimately, you do not face cancer alone, and just as your family can count on you to guide them through your journey, you can incorporate their support along the way. You will form resilient bonds with your children as you traverse the road of survivorship together.

9

Managing Your Relationship and Cancer

A Partner Makes You a Mother—and a Survivor

Motherhood profoundly shapes the identity of many women. Whether you raise your children with a partner or on your own, caring for your family remains a central responsibility. Even when you are healthy, you likely depend on a partner for support and sharing the workload. When cancer enters your life, you must lean on this person even more to share the responsibilities of raising your children. Indeed, a partner might be a boyfriend or girlfriend, or a husband or wife who joins you on your journey of parenting and healing. Because just as cancer becomes part of your daily life, it also becomes part of your marriage or partnership.

Honestly, I'm not sure what I would have done without my husband in my cancer and adult CF journey. We worked hard together to tackle the extreme health challenges that had befallen me, but it was far from smooth sailing. Cancer strains even the strongest relationships. Even the non-cancer problems you tackle together seem more prominent, complex, and challenging. All while you feel vulnerable and weak—precisely why you need your partner even more.

"I was just let go," Alex blurted out when I answered the phone one morning after dropping the kids at school.

"Let go?" I asked, surprised, "What do you mean 'let go'?" Even though I was pretty certain I knew what he meant. His company had been the target of a corporate takeover for months, but we felt it wouldn't impact my husband's job. How could it? I had cancer—there was no room in our lives for him to lose his job on top of everything else.

"I got fired," Alex continued. "Listen, I can't talk now because I have to leave the building. They're taking my company cell phone in a minute, so I'll see you when I get home."

"Wait. Slow down. What are you talking about?" I asked, still mentally trying to grasp what Alex said.

"The organization was sold today and the new owners want all senior managers gone. I'll see you when I get home," he repeated, then hung up.

I stood holding my cell phone in disbelief. It all seemed like some horrendous joke—first cancer, then adult cystic fibrosis, and now this.

The first day after Alex's layoff, I sat in the kitchen and watched him walk briskly by me dressed for work. With his pressed khakis and starched, button down shirt, I half expected him to grab his briefcase and car keys and drive off. Instead, he marched toward our home office with an intense look, barely noticing me. Clearly, there would be no day off for this guy, even without a job.

When I gently inquired what (the hell) he was doing, Alex turned to me, confused.

"What do you mean?" he asked. "I'm going to start looking for a job," pointing to the office door.

"Right this minute? Dressed in your khakis? Don't you want to take a day off to process what happened?" I asked.

He turned back toward the office, ignored me, and kept walking. Immediately, I knew this unemployment period would not be easy. A wife with two life-threatening diseases and three young daughters understandably drove enormous stress. This drill continued for months—the focused walk through the kitchen each morning to our home office, concern etched on his face. Selfishly, I enjoyed having him around the house, even with his mind elsewhere. It kept my mind off my health, the precise thing driving Alex's worry.

Months later, after countless interviews with multiple companies, my husband's job search resulted in a promising role—the only role—in another city. He received a career-defining, dream job offer that felt too hard to turn down. The prospect seemed crazy, but even I knew we needed his job stability and, most importantly, health insurance.

Weeks later, Alex and I flew from Atlanta to St. Louis to look at possible homes and schools for the girls. Only hours into the trip, I knew I didn't have the fortitude to move our family. I refused to uproot our children from the classmates they depended on, my support system of friends and neighbors, and, most importantly, the cadre of doctors overseeing my care. We had big decisions to make for this position that would last two years.

After weeks of discussion and much trepidation, Alex accepted the job and began commuting each week, leaving every Monday morning and returning Thursday night. It's an understatement to say his new position and weekly departures scared me. Deep down, I knew it offered our family the best opportunity, and it was me who chose not to move. However, the anxiety of managing nearly everything alone as the primary parent in the house with limited help felt overwhelming. I wanted to believe that even with cancer, I could morph into a fearless warrior capable of juggling *motherhood while caring for myself and my kids as a semi-single parent. But, as a fragile shell of my former self, this person never materialized. Cancer had sucked my energy and ability to rise to the occasion to serve the family. My old Superwoman self had left the building.*

Cancer can be so aggravating. It strips you of the confidence motherhood breeds and the I-got-this mindset. I hated being dependent on my spouse, but cancer didn't care. I desperately wanted to be that woman: Husband takes a high-powered job in a new city and leaves his wife to care for the kids during the week? No problem! Manage the house and pay the bills? Check. Schedule social plans and family bonding activities for when he comes home each weekend? Done. All while managing cancer and adult CF? I got it.

None of that happened.

Instead, my cesspool of bitterness and anger spilled over into everything. I no longer felt capable of juggling all the balls our children required. Far from being a selfish and distant father, Alex did all he could to help raise our girls from afar. He suffered intense guilt not being able to help in person and hated the impact it was having on all of us. The experience pried open the small cracks that exist in every marriage. Except ours turned into vast chasms of pain and frustration, pushing the outer limits of our marriage. Therapy, a lot of therapy, became our salvation.

Ironically, Alex's new role evolved into a blessing in disguise for me. While he worked hard to support our family, the experience made me stronger and, you guessed it, more self-sufficient. Alex couldn't be a caregiver for the children and me while working a high-powered job in another city. And, while I often railed against him for the intense strain the situation placed on us, I learned to rely on myself even more. I turned to my Tribe, babysitters, and friends to help pick up the physical and emotional slack during the week. I managed the many facets of my health situation independently and grew more reliant and confident in my abilities. I repeatedly told myself: *I'm battling leukemia and cystic fibrosis, going to all my doctor appointments, managing my treatments, and raising my family with my husband in another city? High-five for me.* Perhaps you will discover the same thing—your partner's support might be enough to get you through, but not everything you need.

Managing your relationship with cancer and your partner might mean letting go of many expectations of what your partner should or shouldn't do for you. While I found the inner strength to care for myself with my husband away, it didn't mean I turned inward completely. On the contrary, becoming more self-reliant helped me enjoy my time with Alex more when he returned each weekend. I learned I needed Alex for specific, non-family-related things. He helped me escape my cancer-focused mindset by going out socially or planning a short vacation without the kids to give me a much-needed break. I won't lie; reaching this point took a long time. But, I was better for it.

CANCER'S IMPACT ON YOUR RELATIONSHIP

Cancer will shine a bright light on the tremendous importance and power of a team approach to your disease. Indeed, your cancer experience is as traumatic for your spouse or partner as it is for you. They also feel anxious, scared, and at times helpless. While you're the one living with the disease, they, too, harbor fears—although they might struggle to express them as openly as you do. Your spouse or partner might attempt to appear brave and refrain from letting their guard down in front of you, which makes it doubly challenging for them. Recognizing how to support one another proves crucial.

Once again, I know you're thinking, *But I'm the one with cancer! You told me to be self-sufficient!* Yes, and you may even find it hard to be taken care of by someone you love. You're a strong woman; everyone relies on you to manage nearly everything. Even so, the earlier you understand how to support each other, the more you can build on a solid foundation, no matter what arises.

✓ What Your Cancer Is Like for Your Partner

It would be foolish of me to stand in my husband's shoes and share what he felt and thought during my cancer journey. While Alex and I vowed to be there "in sickness and health," little did we know what might lie ahead. From the earliest hours and days until now, over eighteen years later, he has been on a ride he never signed up for. And yet, thousands of partners face the challenge.

Below is one husband's story of becoming a caregiver to his pregnant wife diagnosed with breast cancer. Chris's powerful story, "Living in the 'Beautiful Mess': One Husband's Caretaking Journey," featured in the National Breast Cancer Foundation's *Stories of Hope* blog, captures what many partners feel and experience.[18]

It was a whirlwind few months for Tamara and Chris. In March 2018, they were celebrating getting married and being newlyweds. A couple of months later, in May, they were overjoyed to learn they were expecting their first child. But while honeymooning together in June, Tamara began to feel a sharp pain in her arm. After undergoing testing, her diagnosis was confirmed: triple negative breast cancer.

Tamara was five months pregnant when she and Chris received the news she had cancer. For Chris, Tamara's diagnosis "...was a blur. My main focus was making sure my wife was ok and trying to figure out how I could be there for her. I didn't know anyone who had gone through this before. It was a huge gut punch. I went into immediate husband mode: How can I support and help?" Because Tamara needed to focus on treatment, Chris was able to "handle everything else, non-treatment wise. I did whatever I could to aid her at the moment. And I still do to this day."

Overnight, Chris went from being a new husband and expectant father to the caregiver of his wife with breast cancer and their unborn child. After initial treatment, doctors determined that Tamara should be induced to give birth two months early so that she could proceed with additional chemo and surgery. After 56 hours of labor, their son Teague was born, weighing five pounds 1 ounce. Almost immediately, Tamara jumped back into treatment, with the new family traveling over four hours to Duke University every day for chemotherapy.

When asked what it was like to adjust to being a new father and a caregiver all at once, Chris shares: "How does anyone cope with all that we've been through without support? I personally owe a lot to God for him sending me such great in-laws, who have been super throughout this whole process. I believe I'm still coping to this day. I have a new definition of so many words now, such as cope, intimacy, love, covenant, reciprocity, longsuffering, and so many more."

Chris shares that while it's important to care for your partner with cancer, it's also important for the caregiver to care for themselves: "Take time for yourself when you can, even if it's five minutes. Read a devotion, do jumping jacks, go outside for some fresh air, or walk to the end of your neighborhood or community. Find something you like to do and try to do it every so often. Get a babysitter, find someone to clean the house, do the laundry, *perhaps cook; if any of those things are possible, invest in them every so often to relieve the stress. At the end of the day, take it one moment at a time."*

Expanding on his role as a caretaker, Chris shares, "You don't want to take things for granted. But we're human, so we can get caught up in emotions. I try to think: Let me be cool. Let me figure out how I can best serve. I don't think caretakers get asked a lot about how they're doing. I appreciate when I'm asked, 'How are you doing?' because you do endure a lot. It can be very challenging, but it can also be beautiful. You can still have a beautiful marriage even though you're on a health journey. It's going to take time and take some digging, but don't give up."

✓ **Managing the Emotional Ups and Downs**

Couples must learn how to cope with the emotional ups and downs cancer inflicts on their relationship. The National Cancer Institute (NCI) states, "Some relationships get stronger during cancer treatment. Others are weakened. Nearly all couples feel more stress than usual when cancer occurs." Other relationship stressors include making difficult decisions about cancer treatment, juggling many roles such as childcare, housekeeping, work, and caregiving, and changing their social life and daily routine.[19]

The NCI also highlights that couples express their emotions differently during the stress of cancer. I used to believe my spouse should share my thoughts and feelings on everything related to my diseases. He didn't. Through trial and error, I learned that Alex cared deeply about my health; he just processed it differently than I did. Sound familiar?

Additionally, I discovered—and you will too—that while some prefer discussing issues openly and talking things out, others do not. These differences create tension. You or your partner might focus inward by doing chores, fixing things around the home, or getting out of the house altogether—anything but talk about cancer. Remind yourself that everyone reacts differently to the emotional pain inflicted by your disease. [20]

Interaction with each other sometimes requires more energy than you realize or have the strength to give. Effective communication during these moments is crucial, as relationships can quickly break down under constant strain. Shock and disbelief surrounding your cancer might cause you and your partner to retreat from each other and communicate less, which results in the opposite of what needs to happen. So often, as I went through the motions of caring for the family, attending to my own needs, pondering the next medical appointment, and striving to feel normal, I didn't have much left for my husband.

Here's the truth—never underestimate the value of your partner's presence. A simple yet powerful gesture from a spouse or partner is their willingness to sit with you and listen. Their presence and openness to hear you convey a crucial message of support. I'm not going to lie; my husband struggled with this, and I would guess your partner might also. It's a universal truth that men, in particular, are hard-wired to fix things. I often had to remind Alex to listen, not fix, just listen. Understandably, some couples find it easier to talk about serious issues than others. Only you and your partner know how you feel about this. The National Cancer Institute shares additional ways to improve communication:[21]

➤ **Share the Decisions.** Try including your spouse or partner in treatment decisions whenever possible. Together, you should meet with your oncologist early on to understand your disease, your treatment plan, its side effects, and its impact on you. These interactions will help you plan for your family and determine what decisions must be made to accommodate your needs.

- **Support Each Other**. Everyone wants to feel needed and loved. You may have always been the "strong one" in your family, but now let your loved one help you. And in turn, make sure you support your partner. You can express your gratitude and let your partner or spouse know you understand it's also a tough time for them. Acknowledging your shared challenges will build the bonds to be a better couple and parents.
- **Be Open about Stress**. Some things that cause stress for you and your partner can't be solved immediately, such as waiting for medical results or understanding what might happen next in your treatment. Still, there are times when talking about these things can be helpful. Look at the issues that bother you, such as dealing with the unknown or feeling an unspeakable strain between you. You may want to say up front, "I know we can't solve this today. But I'd like to talk about how it's going and how we feel." Getting things out into the open will help you both. Don't ignore the elephant in the room.
- **Plan Fun**. Engage in activities together that alleviate isolation because fighting cancer can feel lonely. Your dates don't have to be elaborate; it's about spending time together. Go out with friends or cross things off your *Things I'd Love to Do One Day* list together, anything that takes both your minds off cancer. I recall the Sip and Paint class at a local art studio that I wanted to try with my husband as an alternative to our standard dinner and movie date night. Alex sipped wine and painted his way to a masterpiece while my art looked worse than a

toddler's. We laughed the entire evening and forgot about my diseases. Plan fun, and both of you will feel better.

OTHER AREAS IMPACTED BY YOUR CANCER

Just as cancer invades your body, it invades your relationship, seeping into your daily routines, your emotional tenor, your intimacy—even your ability to maintain the commitment you founded at the beginning of your marriage. Cancer can destroy your partnership just as it can your body, so let's discuss it.

✓ **Let's Talk about Sex**
Or not. Maybe we don't need to talk about sex and cancer because the two go together like oil and water. But, given the role sex plays in any healthy relationship, it's hard to ignore. Some of you might be thinking, *Nope! I'm not going there—let's move on* and skip right over this section. I get it.

For months after my diagnosis, I couldn't think about being sexually intimate. I needed other forms of intimacy, such as hand-holding and a reassuring hug, but a romp in bed? No way. Even sex prompted me to reflect on my mortality. Because I didn't know if I would live or die, sex reminded me that my husband might be intimate with someone else one day. Why even think about that, you ask? I don't know. Why do we think about half the crazy things we think about when we have cancer?

There are a host of psychological and physical issues at play when it comes to cancer and sexuality. Women may not feel up to sexual intimacy after surgeries or during chemo and radiation sessions. Each of these can also change the body, impacting aspects of sexual wellness such as body image and sensations. A woman who has had a mastectomy, for instance, might view her body differently.[22] Many women may not feel comfortable with ports, scars, and other discomforts. Our bodies may react to treatment in ways that don't vibe with sexual interaction. In fact, we may be so uncomfortable that we can't even imagine the pleasure we once enjoyed, the pleasure that began our children. As with everything in your cancer journey, you must choose what feels best for you. Don't feel pressure to please other people at the expense of your well-being.

✓ **Love Lost: Cancer and Divorce**

In many instances, couples grow closer during a spouse's cancer journey and emerge from the experience with their relationship intact. Indeed, research shows that a close marriage can dramatically improve a patient's outcome, highlighting their importance.[23] However, not all bonds are strong enough to survive the understandable strain. According to a study published in the journal *Cancer*, a woman with cancer or other serious illness is six times more likely to be separated or divorced soon after receiving her diagnosis than a male patient.[24]

Marriage counselors also state that cancer can damage a marriage or relationship in several ways. *Cure* magazine shares that a cancer diagnosis affects not only how patients see themselves, but also how they view their life and their relationships. In the context of marriage, cancer brings additional pressure, distress and changes to how a couple operates within their relationship. Communication—which may have been difficult before the diagnosis—often suffers further. Additionally, a cancer diagnosis also negatively affects job security, finances, basic family dynamics and more, putting further strain on any partnership.[25]

Various stressors may erupt as a couple works through

cancer and recovery. A diagnosis may have a devastating emotional impact on a spouse. While many partners readily take on the role of caregiver, not all are prepared for the job, which can be physically and mentally exhausting. Some who are unwilling to face the challenges choose to leave the relationship.[26] Other significant stressors might be finances—especially if money was an issue before the diagnosis. Or there may be resentment on the part of the caregiver. Although they may not directly express their feelings to the patient, those emotions can fester and manifest in more subtle ways. Add children to this combustible mix, and you can understand why marriages suffer when a mom has cancer.[27]

Fortunately, there are ways for couples in crisis (and my husband and I saw our fair share of crises) to keep their relationship strong during cancer treatment and recovery. Foremost, counselors say, is to maintain open lines of communication. Don't hesitate to see a therapist together or alone. Partners should also seek other outside support, such as a support group to help them deal with the stress of their partner's health, their career, and their own emotions.[28] Recognize these options could be difficult for your partner, especially considering family responsibilities and finances are already stretched thin.

✓ **Cancer and the Single Mom**

Being a single mother diagnosed with cancer might feel like the cruelest double whammy. Everyday tasks such as cooking, cleaning, buying groceries, and taking the kids to school can be a struggle—single motherhood or not. Making ends meet with copays and prescriptions and finding childcare for numerous doctor's appointments likely generates financial stress. And if a single mother cannot work, savings might evaporate quickly. With all the pressure of managing your diagnosis and treatment as a single parent, how do you keep your household running and yourself sane? It *is* possible. Surviving cancer as a single parent will demonstrate your courage, vulnerability, and determination—valuable traits for your children to see and model.

Likely, the two most significant areas in which you will need support will be childcare and finances. Many nonprofit organizations assist single mothers in making caring for themselves and their children more manageable. Search the internet for financial, housing, and child support resources in your area. If you're wary about asking too much of friends and family, some cancer care organizations offer transportation assistance, meal delivery, and housecleaning help. Single mothers undoubtedly have to walk a far different journey than their married counterparts surviving cancer, but they possess the same strength and resilience. It's about tapping into that familiar reserve of strength in all of us and having the courage to ask for help.

KEY REFLECTIONS

Cancer can threaten to take over your entire life, including your relationship with your partner. Remembering why the two of you elected to embark on a life-long journey in the first place might center you and help you find the impetus to sustain the most intimate relationship you have. Your partner—no matter how that person deals with your diagnosis and treatment—can be a sustaining force in your cancer journey. That person can lend an ear or a hand in crucial times. Treat them with as much compassion and appreciation as you're able, even in your lowest moments.

Just as you have navigated countless decisions together during your marriage—caring for your children and managing the responsibilities of parenting and adulthood—learn to share the challenges of your cancer journey. And, while single or divorced mothers must face their journey alone, learning to find support from other areas (your Tribe, family, or community) will strengthen you in unimaginable ways.

10

Cancer and the Working Mom

Balancing Your Professional Career, Your Personal Life, and Your Disease

Balancing the responsibilities of motherhood with life's other demands is no easy feat. It comes with unique challenges and joys, especially regarding your work. Whether you work full-time, part-time, or stay at home to raise your children, your dedication to your family extends far beyond any "workplace" boundaries. When cancer enters the picture, it adds complexity that affects all mothers, stay-at-home or working, and demands careful planning.

Before leukemia, I believed I had formulated the perfect plan to sequence my career and raise my children. After building my marketing career, I planned to have children and work from home in an ideal consulting role, setting my own hours while raising them. I imagined working while the kids were in school, arranging after-school activities and babysitters to carve out more time for my business in the afternoons. I thought my biggest challenge would be finding suitable childcare to cement this grand scheme of mine.

Indeed, just before my diagnosis, my career "plan" was in operation as I consulted from home, albeit far less than I had anticipated. My three young daughters demanded most of my time, forcing me to make thoughtful decisions about how much I worked and when. When CML and adult CF blew up my life, I put my career on indefinite hold.

Years later, as my physical and mental health stabilized, I cautiously ventured into freelance work. I was excited to reconnect with this part of myself and reenter the professional world. However, as I endeavored to build a client base and establish a stable business, I felt a nagging sense that piecemeal freelance work wasn't how I wanted to spend my time. Armed with a new appreciation of life, I knew I needed a change, even if I wasn't sure what that change would be.

Clouds drifted below the airplane as the azure-blue sky turned pink and lavender with the setting sun. Flying home to Atlanta from MD Anderson Cancer Center in Houston, where I had yearly check-ups with a leading CML oncologist, I felt elated as I replayed my doctor's words from that morning, "You have achieved remission." An overwhelming sense of relief consumed me as I recalled the years of intense stress, wondering if and when my chemotherapy medication would control my disease. It took me seven years to reach remission. Was it a cure? No, but my bloodstream no longer showed any signs of leukemia. My oncologist informed me that there were likely still undetectable traces of leukemic cells lingering in my bone marrow, but not enough to pose a threat. I had to continue my oral medication as a safeguard. While not out of the woods, I could see the edge of the forest.

Watching the sunset outside the airplane window, I thought of the other patients I saw in the leukemia clinic that morning. They came from all over the world to MD Anderson seeking hope—a cure, maybe, but more likely hope that they, too, might reach remission. I knew some never would.

I Can't Have Cancer, I Have Carpool!

Despite my happy news, I wondered about the mothers with leukemia who, perhaps due to life circumstances, couldn't afford the same specialized medication I had received. What would happen to them? Would they survive CML without the same treatment? Unlikely. What would happen to their children without a loving mother? Elation over my remission and survivor's guilt swirled interchangeably like the winds beneath the plane. I wondered what I could do to pay my good fortune forward. Surely, I thought, there must be a global health or humanitarian organization that could use my help.

At that moment, flying thirty thousand feet above the ground, a light bulb of career clarity flashed brightly. I wondered how I could help people, namely mothers, facing challenging health situations. I figured there must be nonprofits that assist disadvantaged women with cancer, and other diseases, worldwide. Determined to find them, I opened my laptop and began searching. My heart soared as I researched and pondered new career opportunities.

Career planning might be the last thing on your mind following a diagnosis. An avalanche of mind-bending emotions and immediate healthcare decisions might trump thoughts about your work. Your job might be in full swing when you learn you have cancer, forcing you to reorient your life while undergoing treatment. If you were forced to stop working due to your health, deciding when and how to restart your career can be challenging. For some women, it may take days or weeks to return to your role; for others, it may be a year or more. Maybe you want to stop working altogether to be with your children. Perhaps you do not have this luxury and must resume your career—staying home is not an option. Whatever your situation, cancer injects uncertainty at every turn.

Elizabeth Hodges

CANCER—THE GREAT WORK CLARIFIER

According to World Health Organization estimates, over 1.5 million working-age women in the US live with cancer. It impacts all aspects of their work, including how they perform their jobs, interact with coworkers and clients, and their future career prospects.[29] Many diagnosed women and mothers may continue working to avoid losing their income or position. For others, work might be beneficial for the mental distraction and sense of purpose it offers. Indeed, the American Cancer Society shares that 69 percent of cancer survivors said that maintaining a work routine helped them through recovery. [30]

Fortunately, with advancements in cancer treatment, millions of women continue to work. The experience, however, might generate various emotions, reactions, and internal conflict. You might find yourself asking, *Why now? My career is thriving. How can I possibly manage all this?*

What is the best way to deal with this conflict while remaining present in your work and children's lives? How do you tell coworkers or your manager that you have cancer when you can barely wrap your head around it yourself? There is no set formula, but here are some considerations to help you navigate your career, personal life, and disease:

✓ **Decide Who to Tell (Or Not)**

Should you decide to continue working during cancer, you do not have to inform your employer. Privacy might be your preference as you come to terms with your condition and prefer to keep it to yourself. Remember, the Americans with Disabilities Act doesn't require patients to disclose their diagnosis.

However, you may decide to tell your manager if you feel physically and emotionally drained from work while managing your health and home life. Alternatively, your appearance could draw attention to your disease, making it difficult to avoid telling people. Remember to share what you know about your treatment plan at the time and alert your employer that things could change later.

You might discuss your diagnosis with coworkers, so they appreciate the challenges you're facing and how to support you in the workplace. Help colleagues understand what cancer means for working mothers. Some could feel uncomfortable about your disease and its impact on work life.[31] They want to help but don't know how. Be as open as you feel comfortable.

✓ **Learn to Accept a Career Pause (At Least for Now)**

Maybe your career will continue with no disruption. Your treatment may leave you feeling less than stellar, but you can continue in your role. But for some, continuing to work isn't an option. You might choose paid time off during treatment or utilize the Family and Medical Leave Act (FMLA), which allows eligible employees to take unpaid, job-protected leave.[32]

Accepting a career pause may fuel frustration about the totality of your situation. It could be temporary or last for years. Frankly, you don't know what will happen. Speak to a career coach or mentor about your feelings. Be open and honest; these advisors might surprise you with an alternate view of your situation. They might offer the advice you need to hear that you, your health, and your family take center stage for now.

✓ **Lose Your Fear of What Might Happen**

You cannot control how your employer will react if you decide to share your news. I decided to tell my manager about my chronic leukemia years after my diagnosis. I wanted to be honest about my health from the beginning, yet I feared it would impact my ability to get promoted. But, when an annual team meeting required me to share a hotel room with a colleague to help the nonprofit defray costs, I knew it was time to inform my manager of my situation. I could not possibly have shared a hotel room. Leukemia and adult cystic fibrosis required me to take medicines at prescribed times of day and perform maintenance exercises on my lungs with a machine to keep them clear. I needed privacy and a calm environment free from distraction at the end of the day. The timing just felt right.

Sharing my health status generated a lot of personal anxiety, but ultimately, the conversation went well. My boss expressed concern and empathy and worked with me to get the hotel accommodations I needed. Do I think sharing my situation hindered my ability to get promoted in the long run? I'll never know because I later changed jobs, but I do not regret my decision.

Cancer Today magazine reports that many patients are unsure how to discuss their cancer diagnosis with their employer, often experiencing a great deal of fear—fear of not being supported, of being dismissed from their role, or of being supported but perceived differently, which could cause them to miss out on opportunities for professional growth or advancement.[33] However, as more women stay on the job through treatment, work has become a topic for patients, their employers, and oncology teams to consider. Working mothers must understand their rights and discuss their desire to work with their doctors so they know what will and will not be possible to do. Equally, don't assume you can't take a leave of absence and pause your job. Later, you might regret the decision.[34] Bottom line, stay informed of your options, rights, and don't be fearful.

✓ **Life Is Not a Competition**

It's hard to avoid feeling envious of seemingly healthy

mothers, especially those you work with. You juggle so much while in treatment, which adds extra mental and physical effort that others do not have to bear. During work hours, I wanted my mind to mirror that of my coworkers, free from the constant swirl of worry that cancer brings. Though I tried not to question my fate, I found it challenging not to gaze at other working women and crave their cancer-free work lives. I often grew competitive and pushed myself more to prove my point: *Cancer can't stop me; I'm just as good as she is.* I laugh now at the absurdity of this.

Over time, cancer gradually taught me that I wasn't competing with anyone—not as a mother or a working professsional. Instead, I chose to be a role model for my children, an emblem of how to face adversity head-on. I could work and raise my family, even with cancer. Remind yourself that your exemplary work as a stay-at-home mother or a working mom belongs to you and no one else. It is your life to live and not a competition. Your resilience in the face of adversity should rule the day—each and every day.

✓ **What Do You Really Want?**

One of cancer's unexpected "gifts" is a heightened focus on your desires and career aspirations. Perhaps cancer will fuel an insatiable desire to achieve your life and career goals with gusto. Or it might take time to realize what you want fully. Do you prefer more time with your children in a part-time role? A promotion you have long strived for? Armed with an understanding that life is fleeting, you might double down on what you want to accomplish professionally.

Many survivors see cancer as an opportunity to change careers entirely. Maybe you finally want to be your own boss. Ask yourself whether your work brings you joy. Do you enjoy your daily role, industry, and colleagues? Perhaps your job is more of a distraction from your diagnosis than a source of happiness. Maybe you want to prove that you've still got it, and cancer ignites a desire to stay in the game. Whatever the case, listen to the quiet voice within you that reveals your deepest desires.

✓ **Make Your Job Work For YOU**

Now might be the best time to structure your work precisely how you want. When I reentered the workforce, I was fortunate to have part-time employment. This arrangement allowed me to conserve the energy needed to work and raise my daughters while managing my diseases. I know many women do not have this option.

But, even if part-time work is not an option, ask yourself how to structure your job to serve you best. Talk with your manager about the times of day that feel most productive for you during and after treatment. If your role and responsibilities still feel too demanding, ask yourself if a less stressful position might serve you better. This request is not a failure or demotion but a concerted effort to craft a career that helps you navigate a challenging time. Caring for yourself personally and professionally is the right decision. In truth, there are no wrong decisions—just those that help you conquer cancer on your terms.

Now that you understand the personal conflicts cancer inflicts on your career and things for you to consider, how do you make the nuts and bolts of your family, and your career, fit together if you do return to your job? It's a work-life balancing act like no other.

CANCER AND THE WORKING MOM: THE ULTIMATE BALANCING ACT

Working mothers expertly juggle numerous responsibilities. Balancing a career and family presents enough challenges, but adding a major hurdle like cancer can feel overwhelming. Managing work-life balance while dealing with your disease can evoke a range of feelings, from frustration and disbelief to pride and confidence in knowing you're doing your best to handle it all. Whatever your reason for continuing to work while undergoing cancer treatment is commendable, give yourself credit for not giving up. Remember that much of your balancing act as a working mother will remain the same. The systems you put in place to manage your family and career before cancer will still function, but now you must add managing your disease to the mix.

I love this abbreviated article by *Wildfire* magazine founder and editor-in-chief April Johnson Stearns, who details her experience as a working mother with a young child. Her article, "Adding 'Patient' to the Work-Life Balance: Moms with Cancer Under 40," discusses how life, career, and parenting collide when cancer enters the picture.[35]

When I was diagnosed with breast cancer, my daughter was just three years old. She had not yet started preschool. My husband and I shared in her care: I worked from home for several hours each day and then we switched: I took over caring for our daughter while my husband went off to work. Often I would work through my daughter's naps, and again in the middle of the night after she'd gone to bed. There was always work to be done. As the primary breadwinner, I felt compelled to work as much as possible while also striving to be as hands-on as possible for my daughter. Even when I went on business trips, which was frequent, my husband took time off work so he and my daughter could come along. I recall many times when I would dash to our hotel room for a quick nursing session before fixing my makeup, straightening my nylons, and dashing back downstairs to work.

And then I was diagnosed with stage III breast cancer.

Although I stopped traveling, I did continue to work through my year of cancer treatment (I didn't fully appreciate how hard this was until after the chemo fog finally started to lift!). I had to take a step back from some of the parenting I was doing, and that was incredibly hard for me because this really scary thing was happening to our family. I really didn't know if I was going to survive it, and I didn't want to traumatize my daughter further by pulling back from her during this crisis.

We were accustomed to seeing each other all the time, every day. Even while I was working, I was only working a hallway away and often had one ear out for her cries. For all intents and purposes, she was my number one priority. If I'm being honest, it was probably my child, then work, then my husband, and then myself way down at the bottom of the totem pole. But cancer. Cancer reshuffled the order. Overnight, I had to move myself—my body—to the top of the list.

Concerns about the impact of your cancer on you, your children, and your significant other only add more stress to your complicated decision to keep working. Perhaps you don't have a choice as a single mother or the primary breadwinner. Whatever the case, there are ways to make the transition more manageable or at least tolerable while undergoing treatment.

Here are some issues to consider to help transition to working while undergoing treatment or when returning to work:

- ✓ **How Will Your Treatment Plan Constrain or Interrupt Your Work?**

Work closely with your medical team to understand the timing and side effects of your treatment regimen, as some effects may not appear right away. Fatigue, nausea, or hair loss might immediately impact you or take longer to develop. Discuss the timing of treatments—whether daily, weekly, or monthly—and how much time to budget for each. Knowing these details will help you plan your return to work and manage expectations.

Some moms can utilize the Family Medical Leave Act (FMLA) to keep their jobs through cancer treatment, allowing them to take time off if needed. Research your rights regarding unpaid leave, the US Department of Labor recommendations, and what benefits your state provides.[36] Many people don't realize they can take FMLA in segments—for a week or even a day at a time—rather than all at once.

✓ **What Should You Do If Your Employer Is Acting Discriminatorily?**

Unfortunately, women with cancer sometimes face discrimination in the workplace. Cancer still carries a stigma in society, and people do not understand how the disease affects daily life. Mothers with cancer may face workplace discrimination issues, such as being passed over for promotions and wage increases while also being overlooked for career opportunities. Women diagnosed with cancer are more likely to be fired from their jobs than women without a history of cancer. And one in four report that they were discriminated against at work due to their diagnosis.[37]

Remember that you have rights. Familiarize yourself with the Equal Employment Opportunity Commission (EEOC) and prevailing anti-discrimination laws. If someone discriminates against you, they must understand the implications of their actions and how destructive those behaviors can be. Again, research your rights and what to do if you feel you are being discriminated against due to your disease. Federal protections (Americans with Disabilities Act or ADA) also exist for employees with short- or long-term disabilities, making it illegal to discriminate against someone based on their cancer diagnosis.[38]

KEY REFLECTIONS

Many mothers with cancer face decisions concerning their professional life in addition to all of the disruptions they must manage in the lives of their children, families, relationships, and "regularly scheduled programming." Navigating cancer's effect on your work life has great value because it helps you gain insight into its broader impact on your overall life. Many women found great purpose and definition through their careers before they became mothers. Becoming a mom deepened the sense of identity you developed when you first set out to support yourself and contribute to your family.

English novelist Joseph Conrad famously wrote, "I don't like work... but I like what is in work—the chance to find yourself. Your own reality—for yourself, not for others..."[39] Discovering who you uniquely are allows you to be your best self—as a partner, a mother, and in every role you play. By finding the balance between cancer and work, you can continue to be your best self in all areas of your life.

11

The Journey Forward

*An Unknowable Road,
but You Have What It Takes*

Cancer teaches you to expect the unexpected. While nothing can fully prepare you for life's curveballs, your experience teaches invaluable lessons in resilience. You learn that even after overcoming cancer, other significant life events and health issues may arise. As a survivor, you know you face ongoing follow-up to ensure your disease remains in remission or that you stay cancer-free. How do you manage this unpredictability when you feel you've already faced the worst? The first step involves accepting that this will be your journey.

Over the years, I've grappled with how I could have been diagnosed with two life-threatening chronic diseases within six weeks of each other. It felt unjust, like being struck by lightning twice in the same storm. No amount of preparation could have equipped me for even one of these battles, let alone two. I remember naively thinking after my CML diagnosis, *What are the chances of getting another disease in my lifetime?* It only took six weeks to find out, and my life has never been the same. Adult cystic fibrosis taught me the challenges of what can follow cancer.

And yet, I know situations like this happen all the time. People get two or three types of cancer and various diseases in a lifetime. You may know some people who have experienced this yourself. Ruth Bader Ginsberg, former Supreme Court justice, is a shining example of a survivor who, before her death, survived three different cancers over twenty years. In 1999, Ginsburg was diagnosed and successfully treated for colon cancer at the age of thirty-six. In 2009 came a new diagnosis: early-stage pancreatic cancer, discovered during regular screenings for her first cancer. Finally, at the age of eighty-five, doctors surgically removed two tumors from Ginsberg's lungs along with a new malignancy discovered in her pancreas.[40]

I can't imagine battling three different types of cancer over twenty years. Just when you think you've overcome one challenge, another diagnosis forces you to gather the strength and courage to fight again. Ginsburg showed remarkable bravery, proving that life must go on, refusing to let cancer define her.

As a woman, cancer is likely to be just one of several health challenges you may face, including the lingering effects of your disease. Many side effects from cancer treatment improve once treatment ends. Sometimes, side effects linger and cause long-term problems. Or, issues may not show up for months or even years later. These are called late effects, and they can take many forms. And just like the side effects you experienced during treatment, late effects vary from person to person.[41]

When discussing your post-treatment health plan with your oncologist, ask about potential late effects to monitor.

I Can't Have Cancer, I Have Carpool!

These may include, among others, bone or memory loss, endocrine or hormone problems, hearing loss, vision changes, ongoing fatigue, heart and lung issues, or lymphedema.[42] While you will likely not encounter many of these, expecting late effects or other long-term health issues will make them easier to face if they happen. Frustrating, right? Welcome to your life post-cancer. Never, however, let the thought of potential future health issues diminish your joy over reaching survivorhood.

SURVIVING CANCER—AGAIN

Let's address what might concern you even more than late effects: the fear of your disease returning or developing a second cancer. No matter how long it has been since you completed treatment, there may be moments when you fear recurrence. While every lump, nodule, or odd sensation won't necessarily be cancer, it's often where your mind goes first. Here is the good news: only 1 to 3 percent of survivors develop a second cancer different from their initial disease. The risk level is low, and more survivors are living longer thanks to improvements in treatment.[43] Still, just thinking about the possibility of a second cancer can be stressful. Fear of recurrence can be just as great. These same fears plagued me for years.

"Your PCR is now .04," my oncologist shared in a somewhat relaxed tone during a routine follow-up phone call in August 2023. PCR, or polymerase chain reaction, is a routine blood test to determine the level of leukemia in my body. Just eighteen months earlier, I had stopped taking my oral chemotherapy medicine, Gleevec, which I took daily to keep my CML under control. After years of favorable test results showing I was in deep

135

remission, my doctor suggested I discontinue the medication to see if the cancer would return or, more importantly, if I might be cured.

"As we discussed multiple times, we knew this might happen once you stopped Gleevec," my oncologist continued in our call. "Your leukemia has reached detectable levels in your bloodstream again. I'm sorry."

My heart broke. For years before stopping Gleevec, my blood tests consistently came back as "Undetectable," showing no trace of leukemia. However, the doctors could not confirm if I was officially cured. The only way to validate it would be to stop taking the medication. My reluctance to stop Gleevec was driven by one thing — my children. As irrational as it seemed, the mental comfort I gained from knowing my disease was under control while taking that pill was more valuable to me than facing the uncertainty of a possible cure. I couldn't bear the risk, let alone the fear and mental torment, of being off the very thing keeping me alive while raising my twins in their final years of high school. But as they approached graduation and with my oldest daughter already out of college, I decided the time had come. I began to believe a cure might be possible, even for me.

And so, in March 2022, sixteen years after my diagnosis and in close consultation with my oncologist, I stopped taking Gleevec. Sadly, just a year and a half later, I received the news no one wanted to hear. My cancer had returned.

"OK, so what does this mean?" I asked my doctor as our call continued, rubbing my forehead nervously. A wave of sadness and defeat washed over me. While I knew my chances of staying off Gleevec and being cured for life were 50/50, I wanted to be one of the lucky ones. Tired of taking a daily chemo pill, I desperately hoped to put cancer behind me.

"Well, as you know, there are several new, stronger medications that we can try that will likely put you back into deep remission very quickly," my oncologist said, trying to sound hopeful.

I Can't Have Cancer, I Have Carpool!

"Mmhmm," I mumbled, half listening. My heart sank further as tears began to fall. For over a year, being off my medication had been life-changing. The subtle but persistent side effects I experienced vanished: no more fatigue, gastrointestinal problems, headaches, mood swings, weight gain, facial swelling, or thinning hair. My energy returned to a level I had long forgotten.

Most importantly, I felt happier. Only after I stopped Gleevec did I realize how much it had impacted my overall well-being. I felt cured both physically and mentally of leukemia. Of course, I still had adult cystic fibrosis to contend with, but I'd take it.

"Will the side effects from the medicine come back again?" I inquired with trepidation, knowing the answer before I even asked.

"Yes, probably. But, they will dissipate over time like before," my oncologist answered, trying to find something to lift my spirits. "Look, your PCR numbers are still very low. There's no danger of your leukemia getting out of control. We just need to keep it that way."

It sounded so simple! Just go back on your medication, and all will be well again! But I wouldn't be well. I still had cancer and likely would for the rest of my life. Yes, it would be chronic and manageable, but not cured. Once more, I had to dig deep and keep fighting. My short, glorious taste of a cure was over. Of course, I knew I should have been thankful I could simply take a pill to treat the return of my disease. But I wasn't. The psychological blow of having cancer reemerge hit me hard. And because there is no cure for adult cystic fibrosis, I was right back where I started—still battling CML and CF. Amor fati, I told myself, amor fati.

Concerns about recurrence or second cancers come naturally. Managing these fears begins with knowing that you survived once and can do it again. Begin by employing the skills you learned as a survivor the first time. While the disappointment will be great, remain steadfast in the practices outlined in this book to ensure you move forward and fight for the most important person and people in the world—you and your family.

YOU HAVE ALL IT TAKES

The familiar notes of "Pomp and Circumstance" swelled in the amphitheater and floated across the warm summer air. Blue graduation gowns and tassels on caps swayed in unison with the music as the students marched in, smiling and proud. I craned to see my twin daughters among the three hundred graduating seniors. Spotting them, I waved to get their attention; I wanted my girls to see me. Whether they were eight or eighteen, I wanted them to feel my presence as I cheered them on one final time. Just a year earlier, my oldest daughter had graduated from college, filling us with immense pride as we celebrated her hard work and achievements. Now, it was the twins' turn, and soon, they all would be off on their own.

The school principal began the ceremony by encouraging parents to celebrate and honor the moment. "You did it! You have prepared your children, and they are ready!" she said, referring to the start of their journey into adulthood. Listening to the principal's words, I wondered if I was ready. Hadn't I hoped, wished, and prayed to reach this moment? Joy and sadness swept over me, blending into one bittersweet feeling.

For weeks before graduation, I challenged myself to recall memories of their childhood. What was the school play in fifth grade? What age did they get braces? I tried to picture them playing violin, drums, and piano, desperately wanting to remember the exact sizes of their little hands. Why does time fly when our children are slipping away—no longer holding our hand but grasping a new future?

I knew I kept replaying these moments in my mind as a way of saying, "Screw you, cancer. You didn't stop me." Even if some

I Can't Have Cancer, I Have Carpool!

memories were hazy, together they formed a beautiful tapestry of survival. That evening, I felt a profound sense of personal achievement. Together with my husband, we succeeded in raising our daughters, caring for them while I fought cancer and CF, and preparing them for life as adults.
I. Made. It.

What began as a prayer for more time to watch my children grow up sixteen years prior became a determination to do whatever it took to survive. I found empowerment and strength in motherhood, using it to regain a sense of control by focusing on what I knew. The strength my daughters saw in me then, and still see today, came from an inner fortitude forged out of necessity. Like you, I had to adapt both my life and my approach to motherhood to meet the demands of my situation. I became a resourceful, adaptive, and loving mother while also confronting cancer. It wasn't always easy or graceful.

I now realize that my children came to see me as the strongest person they knew because they witnessed me prioritize being their mom above all else. I wasn't always like that—I had other ambitions, like working and pursuing personal interests. But cancer taught me to focus on one thing at a time, like driving carpool. You can't think about cancer when you're focused on getting your kids where they need to be. Carpool became a lifeline—a straightforward task that provided a break from the complexity and fear of what might come next.

Cancer begins as a frightening sojourn to a place where you do not know what will happen. It spits you out as a changed person on the other side of your journey, wiser and resilient. Armed with this wisdom, you learn to use motherhood as your anchor to reality because so much of your experience is unknown. As you adjust to your life with cancer as a mother and all its complexities, remember that nothing is permanent. You will move past this, one way or another, and be stronger for it. Along the way, don't forget:

- ✓ **You must become your own cheerleader, advocate, health coach, fitness instructor, therapist, and pharmacist.**

No one will care for you as well as you care for yourself. That is not to say your husband or partner is not the best supporter and fellow journeyman. This is also not to say that people are uncompassionate. They are human. It means you need to take responsibility for knowing everything about your disease and treatment. Though it may be exhausting, overwhelming, and frightening, breaking your condition into manageable pieces helps you regain a sense of control. Yes, share your emotional and physical challenges with people who want to help you, but always remember the buck stops with you. You are the cancer survivor; develop your self-sufficiency to feel empowered and confident.

- ✓ **Find Your Tribe**

Seek out the people you can trust not to judge or feel sorry for you because you never, ever want a pity party on your cancer journey. You want people who will be there—no questions asked, ready to show up and listen. Sometimes, you just want to chat because if you talk about your cancer, One. More. Time. You might snap. Talk to your Tribe about their problems—it takes the focus off you and feels good.

- ✓ **Remember the infinite other resources that exist for mothers with cancer.**

Whether you get assistance directly from your treatment center—and most do offer comprehensive services—or turn to the internet, finding this support is critical. Knowing where to seek and find help should become your superpower. Bonding with other women who share your journey begins with support groups—walking the road with people with similar forms of cancer. There were no local support groups for chronic myelogenous leukemia in my city, but many online. So, I started my own because I wanted to sit face-to-face with people with the same disease. I wanted to see their faces. You can do the same.

- ✓ **Know that you and your family will face many challenges as you adjust to your "new normal."**

Cancer thrusts a lot on families. Take it slow and trust your gut as a mother to know when one of your children struggles with your situation. Again, countless resources exist for families experiencing cancer. Living your new normal will teach you to value your limited time on earth. Seeing the world through a different lens is a gift. My children have seen me work tirelessly to live fully. They have also heard me scream and cry about my health and then pick myself up and keep going. Little did they know I was trying hard to keep moving for them.

- ✓ **Form solid relationships with your doctors, nurses, and anyone in your healthcare orbit.**

Leverage your care team's expertise by seeking their advice on every aspect of your disease. Research your specific type of cancer thoroughly so you can ask well-informed questions and make crucial decisions about your care. This approach will boost your confidence and help you feel like you're gaining ground in understanding your condition. Building this relationship also opens the door to asking personal, non-medical questions. For critical decisions, I never hesitated to ask my doctors, "If you were in my position, with three children, what would you do?" They always gave me an honest answer I could trust.

✓ **Learn to "Jump the Rails."**

Often you don't want to think about your cancer, but it's always there. Whether going for treatments or tests, taking countless medications at specific times of day, or managing the physical and demoralizing side effects of your chemo, you feel like you can never outrun your illness. Many days, you just want to feel normal. You can achieve this by learning to "jump the rails." In your mind, ride the Normal Train, not the Cancer Train. Learn how to act and feel "normal" to the outside world and yourself. Yes, many people know your situation, but many do not. Rather than living and feeling like a cancer patient 24/7, leave it aside.

I understand that it might seem odd to deny your reality, especially if you have visible symptoms of your illness. However, you might see the benefits when you give it a try. Even if you experience physical changes from your disease, most people won't notice them. Do you honestly notice if a woman is wearing a wig or has had a radical mastectomy? I certainly don't. Occasionally, stepping away from your "Cancer Train" and allowing yourself to feel normal, like everyone else, can be incredibly beneficial. Trust me, it will help you stay sane. Your mind can be a powerful force for good.

✓ **Love your fate and the cards you have been dealt.**

It's so easy to feel sorry for yourself, and on many days, it's OK to allow just that. But then, ask yourself if there is a different way to view your cancer. Gratitude certainly has a powerful place in your journey, but what if you could be thankful for your disease? Once diagnosed, try completely accepting and loving your fate—*amor fati*. I would not be the person I am today without cancer. It has become an undeniable part of my life story, so I choose to love it. For many women, this might be a bridge too far. Love the very thing tearing your life apart? If you cannot love your fate, try to find the silver lining. Behind the pain, frustration, loss of self, and all the other shit cancer throws your way, are countless life lessons to be learned.

- ✓ **There might be challenges in your marriage or relationship. Or not.**

From increased responsibilities with your children to intense fear of the unknown, your cancer may affect your relationship due to the sheer stress involved. Luckily, your spouse or partner will likely rise to the occasion and become the Superman or Superwoman you need them to be. But be prepared that they may not. Communication remains critical, and everyone—including you—is entitled to their feelings. Remember, therapy is always one click or phone call away. As I have repeatedly emphasized, counseling during cancer treatment could be exactly what you and your family need.

- ✓ **Live and work the way you want once cancer teaches its innumerable lessons.**

Return to your career, but on your terms if you are able. Once again, maybe you want to stay home with your children. Make the choices that bring you the most happiness and focus on what you love. Don't miss this cancer life lesson—never settle for less in the work that you choose to do. Find your passion and chase it fiercely.

YOUR FINAL CALL TO ACTION

My twin daughters are now in college, the last of my children to leave the nest following their older sister. I marvel at the voyage that brought me to this point. Motherhood guided me through cancer, adult cystic fibrosis, and countless uncertainties, leading me to survivorship. Between oncology appointments and carpool lanes, I learned that surviving cancer isn't just about beating the disease—it's about showing up every single day for the ones who need you most. Including yourself.

Now, it's your turn. Set your sights on your goals, no matter how big or small and pursue them with determination. Let motherhood—or any other passion—be your guide. Embrace your journey, knowing that each day you survive and thrive is a victory.

Above all, remember that you are stronger than you think. Keep moving forward with courage and love, knowing you have everything needed to overcome whatever challenges come your way. I understand some might say this all sounds too simplistic, that driving carpool and motherhood alone aren't enough to keep your mind off cancer. To which I say—really? It might be all you have. Why not focus on the most important job in front of you? You and your family will be richer for it, I promise.

Now, check your watch. Is it time for carpool?

Go.

Acknowledgments

This book is a testament to the love, strength, and resilience of my family, who have been my unwavering source of inspiration throughout this journey. Mia, Lily, and Eliza, you have faced so much with me over the years, and your resilience fills me with pride every day. It is an honor to be your mom. Alex, you are my constant and steadfast partner. Thank you for your encouragement and patience love with this project. I am forever grateful for your sharp editorial insights that guided me to the finish line. I admire you and the incredible family we have built together.

This book would not have been possible without the guidance and belief of Justin Spizman, who encouraged me to "get it done." Thank you for seeing the story in me and leading me to the finish line of this eighteen-year endeavor.

To my dear friend, Professor Leah Hughes, who urged me to "get it right." Thank you for teaching me the craft of storytelling, for your patience, and for the countless conversations that helped shape this book. Your wisdom, support, and friendship have meant the world to me.

A heartfelt thank you to the talented team at BookLogix in Atlanta for making the publishing process both enjoyable and seamless. Your creativity and dedication turned my vision into reality.

And finally, to you, the reader—thank you for choosing to embark on this journey with me. It is my deepest hope that my story and advice offer you comfort, encouragement, and inspiration as you navigate your own path to survivorship.

Endnotes

[1] "Talking to Children and Teenagers," Macmillan Cancer Support, https://www.macmillan.org.uk/cancer-information-and-support/diagnosis/talking-about-cancer/talking-to-children-and-teenagers.

[2] Guy Winch, PhD, "10 Crucial Differences Between Worry and Anxiety... and why you need to know the difference.," Psychology Today, March 14, 2016, https://www.psychologytoday.com/gb/blog/the-squeaky-wheel/201603/10-crucial-differences-between-worry-and-anxiety.

[3] "Signs of Anxiety," Psychology Today, https://www.psychologytoday.com/us/basics/anxiety/signs-of-anxiety.

[4] "Amor Fati: The Formula for Human Greatness Stoic Exercises, Wisdom, and More," Daily Stoic, https://dailystoic.com/amor-fati-love-of-fate/.

[5] "Amor Fati: The Formula for Human Greatness Stoic Exercises, Wisdom, and More," Daily Stoic, https://dailystoic.com/amor-fati-love-of-fate/.

[6] Ashley Melfi, "Jimmy V's ESPY Speech, Annotated," ESPN, https://www.espn.com/espn/feature/story/_/id/24087641/jimmy-v-espys-speech-annotated.

[7] Shah, Binay K et al. "Impact of Parental Cancer on Children." Anticancer research vol. 37,8 (2017): 4025-4028. doi:10.21873/anticanres.11787 (Binay K. Shah, Jeffrey Armaly, and Erin Swieter, "Impact of Parental Cancer on Children," Anticancer Research, August 2017), https://ar.iiarjournals.org/content/37/8/4025.long.

[8] Shah, Armaly, and Swieter, "Impact of Parental Cancer on Children."

[9] Shah, Armaly, and Swieter, "Impact of Parental Cancer on Children."

[10] Shah, Armaly, and Swieter, "Impact of Parental Cancer on Children."

[11] Shah, Armaly, and Swieter, "Impact of Parental Cancer on Children."

[12] Shah, Armaly, and Swieter, "Impact of Parental Cancer on Children."

[13] "When a Parent Has Cancer: the Emotional and Psychosocial Impact," Kesem, https://www.kesem.org/post/when-a-parent-has-cancer-the-emotional-and-psychosocial-impact.

[14] U.S. Department of Health and Human Services National Institutes of Health, "When Your Parent Has Cancer A Guide for Teens," *NIH Publication NO. 12-5734* (The National Cancer Institute 2012), https://www.cancer.gov/publications/patient-education/when-your-parent-has-cancer.pdf.

[15] Shah, Armaly, and Swieter, "Impact of Parental Cancer on Children."

[16] Shah, Armaly, and Swieter, "Impact of Parental Cancer on Children."

[17] Shah, Armaly, and Swieter, "Impact of Parental Cancer on Children."

¹⁸ Stories of Hope "Living in the "Beautiful Mess": One Husband's Caretaking Journey," National Breast Cancer Foundation, Inc., May 18, 2023, www.nationalbreastcancer.org/blog/living-in-the-beautiful-mess-one-husbands-caretaking-journey/.

¹⁹ "Facing Cancer with Your Spouse or Partner," National Cancer Institute, https://www.cancer.gov/about-cancer/coping/adjusting-to-cancer/spouse-or-partner.

²⁰ "Facing Cancer with Your Spouse or Partner," National Cancer Institute.

²¹ "Facing Cancer with Your Spouse or Partner," National Cancer Institute.

²² Cassie Shortsleeve, "How Cancer Changes Your Sex Life—and What You Can Do About It," Yale Medicine, June 9, 2022, https://www.yalemedicine.org/news/sex-intimacy-after-cancer.

²³ Don Vaughan, "Love Lost: The Effects of Cancer on Marriage and Relationships," MJH Life Sciences, October 28, 2021, https://www.curetoday.com/view/love-lost-the-effects-of-cancer-on-marriage-and-relationships.

²⁴ Glantz, Michael J et al., "Gender disparity in the rate of partner abandonment in patients with serious medical illness." Cancer vol. 115,22 (2009): 5237-42. doi:10.1002/cncr.24577

²⁵ Don Vaughan, "Love Lost: The Effects of Cancer on Marriage and Relationships."

²⁶ Don Vaughan, "Love Lost: The Effects of Cancer on Marriage and Relationships."

²⁷ Don Vaughan, "Love Lost: The Effects of Cancer on Marriage and Relationships."

²⁸ Don Vaughan, "Love Lost: The Effects of Cancer on Marriage and Relationships."

29 Mona Jhaveri, "Women with Cancer in the Workplace," MusicBeatsCancer (blog), July 7, 2021, https://musicbeatscancer.org/women-with-cancer-in-the-workplace.

30 Mona Jhaveri, "Women with Cancer in the Workplace."

31 Mona Jhaveri, "Women with Cancer in the Workplace."

32 Family and Medical Leave Act, US Department of Labor, Wage and Hour Division, https://www.dol.gov/agencies/whd/fmla.

33 Leigh Labrie, "The Work-Cancer Balance," Cancer Today, October 1, 2015, https://www.cancertodaymag.org/fall2015/balancing-work-cancer-treatment/

34 Leigh Labrie, "The Work-Cancer Balance."

35 April Johnson Stearns, "Adding 'Patient' to the Work-Life Balance: Moms With Cancer Under 40," https://www.linkedin.com/pulse/adding-patient-work-life-balance-moms-cancer-under-40-april-stearns/.

36 "Cancer in the Workplace and the ADA," US Equal Employment Opportunity Commission, https://www.eeoc.gov/laws/guidance/cancer-workplace-and-ada.

37 Mona Jhaveri, "Women with Cancer in the Workplace."

38 "Cancer in the Workplace and the ADA," US Equal Employment Opportunity Commission.

39 Joseph Conrad, "Heart of Darkness/The Congo Diary," Edited by Owen Knowles (Penguin Classics, 2007), 29.

40 Steven Petrow, "Cancer: Don't Forget That Accolade When It Comes to Ruth Bader Ginsburg's Remarkable Life," STAT News, September 22, 2020, www.statnews.com/2020/09/22/ruth-bader-ginsburg-remarkable-life-cancer-survivor.

41 "Late Effects of Cancer Treatment," National Cancer Institute, https://www.cancer.gov/about-cancer/coping/survivorship/late-effects#second-primary-cancers.

42 "Late and Long Term Effects of Cancer," American Cancer Society, https://www.cancer.org/cancer/survivorship/long-te rm-health-concerns/long-term-side-effects-of-cancer.html.

43 "Second Cancers," Livestrong.org, https://www.livestrong.org/we-can-help/healthy-living-after-treatment/second-cancers.

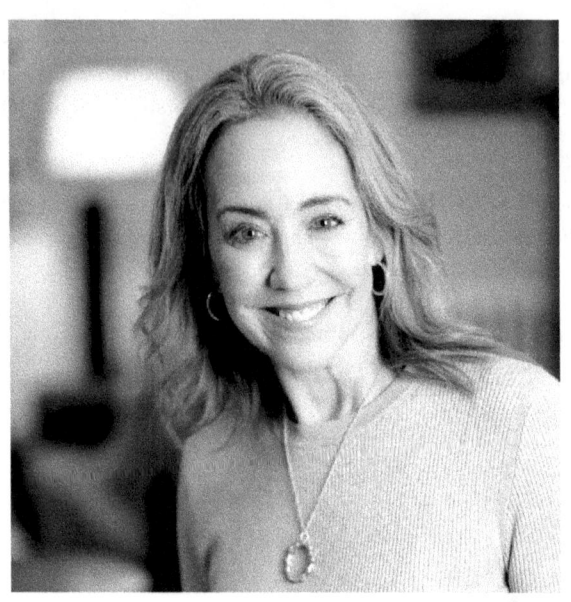

About the Author

Elizabeth Hodges is an eighteen-year leukemia and adult cystic fibrosis survivor. As an accomplished global advertising and marketing executive, she spent her early career working for Fortune 500 companies, including Ogilvy & Mather and GlaxoSmithKline. After her experience with these life-changing diseases, Elizabeth transitioned to working with nonprofits in the public health and education sectors. She is the proud mother of three adult daughters. Elizabeth and her husband split their time between England and Florida, where she continues to write and share her story. *I Can't Have Cancer, I Have Carpool!* is her first book.

www.ingramcontent.com/pod-product-compliance
Lightning Source LLC
Chambersburg PA
CBHW071711020426
42333CB00017B/2227